Pocket Guide to Ayurvedic Healing

Candis Cantin Packard

The Crossing Press
Freedom, California

Copyright © 1996 by Candis Cantin Packard
Cover illustration and design by Victoria May
Book design by Sheryl Karas
Printed in the U.S.A.

*No part of this publication may be reproduced or transmitted in any form or by
any means, electronic or mechanical, including photocopy, recording, or any information storage and retrieval system now known or to be invented, without
permission in writing from the publisher, except by a reviewer who wishes to
quote brief passages in connection with a review written for inclusion in a maga-
zine, newspaper, or broadcast. Contact The Crossing Press, Inc., P.O. Box 1048,
Freedom, CA 95019.*

Cautionary Note: The nutritional information, recipes, and instructions contained within this book are in no way intended as a substitute for medical coun-
seling. Please do not attempt self-treatment of a medical problem without con-
sulting a qualified health practitioner.

    The author and The Crossing Press expressly disclaim any and all liabil-
ity for any claims, damages, losses, judgments, expenses, costs, and liabilities of
any kind or injuries resulting from any products offered in this book by partici-
pating companies and their employees or agents. Nor does the inclusion of any
resource group or company listed within this book constitute an endorsement
or guarantee of quality by the author or The Crossing Press.

Library of Congress Cataloging-in-Publication Data

Packard, Candis Cantin.
    Pocket guide to Ayurvedic healing / Candis Cantin Packard.
       p. cm.
    Includes index.
    ISBN 0-89594-764-1
    1. Medicine, Ayurvedic--Handbooks, manuals, etc. I. Title.
R605.P32   1996
615.5'3--dc20
                                         95-51803
                                         CIP

About the Author

Candis Cantin Packard is a practicing herbalist and teacher of the Ayurvedic healing tradition. She has been applying the principles of Ayurveda to her life and herbal practice for eleven years. She and her husband, Lonnie, have extensive herb gardens at their business and home, EverGreen Herb Garden, in the Sierra Nevada mountains of California, where they grow more than 250 different herbs organically. Candis and Lonnie teach intensive study programs integrating Western herbology with Ayurveda.

I would like to thank my teachers for their inspiration and love: Michael Tierra, for his courageous spirit; Dr. Vasant Lad, for his devotional heart; and David Frawley, for the vision he embraces. And special thanks to my husband, Lonnie, for his steady and gentle love.

TABLE OF CONTENTS

*To the Great Divine Mother
and the green healing plants*

Preface

Ayurveda, the "science of life," is one branch of the ancient Vedic philosophy that has been practiced in India for at least four millennia and is said to have been first "realized" by ancient Seers, or "seekers of truth," who lived in the Himalayas. Ayurveda, developed out of two of the Vedas—the Rig Veda and Atharva Veda—combines physical, psychological, and spiritual therapies in an approach to health that is as relevant to our modern society as it was to the ancient world. Utilizing herbs, proper nutrition, purification and, above all, an affirmative way of living, Ayurveda treats not just the ailment but the whole person, with emphasis on disease prevention rather than the cure of specific symptoms. With the restoration of balance and harmony to the mind and body, the patient can begin to experience the wholeness of life, embarking upon a journey of self-inquiry and self-realization.

Most of our modern methods of diagnosis and treatment are not based on such an integrated understanding of the whole person. Many of the available pharmaceutical preparations and medical procedures merely serve to suppress symptoms, and do not address the lifestyle choices that may be at the root of systemic imbalance. Ayurveda is not a passive form of therapy, but instead asks each individual to take a causative and responsible role in his or her own living and healing process.

As a clinical herbalist, I have found that the Ayurvedic philosophy's holistic vision for living is easily incorporated into a Western cultural matrix, and I have geared the information in this pocket guide to the Western reader. We do not, for example, have to rely exclusively on foreign herbs, which may be hard to obtain, in order to practice Ayurveda. We can practice our Ayurvedic lifestyle and herbal therapies with materials that are readily available, whether grown at home, gathered in the wild or purchased from the local herbalist or health-food store. Therefore, this book will recommend mostly Western herbs, along with some of the more easily obtained East Indian and Chinese herbs.

This guide is designed as a reference book, providing easy access to basic information on Ayurveda and the relevant therapies, focusing on the three constitution types (*doshas*) and on specific lifestyle recommendations. You will also learn about the Ayurvedic system of classifying the different tastes of herbs and other foodstuffs. By understanding the different tastes, or *rasas*, we can experience a deeper understanding of why certain substances are helpful or harmful to our well-being.

Readers who wish to delve deeper into Ayurveda will want to have a look at the Recommended Reading List, as well as at the list of Institutes of Ayurvedic Studies, near the end of the book. In the meantime, I hope you will find the information contained in this brief pocket guide both useful and fascinating.

Introduction

Ayurveda is the medicine of nature, the medicine of life. It does not give us a set of theoretical principles to impose upon our biological functioning. Rather, it seeks to present to the human mind the principles and powers of Nature herself. It teaches us to put into practice Nature's great principles of health and natural living. For this reason it employs the language of nature—an energetic system of the elements and biological humors, a simple yet profound system of correspondences, not a complex scientific, materialistic or biochemical terminology.

—David Frawley, *The River of Life*

The system of healing known as Ayurveda—from the Sanskrit *ayur* ("life" or "longevity") and *veda* ("knowledge" or "wisdom")—helps us to harmonize our minds, bodies, and lifestyles with our spiritual purpose. The language of Ayurveda is based on that which is observable in nature. We experience things as hot or cold, sweet or sour, light or heavy, dry or damp, and so forth. As you go through this booklet, you will find out about the herbs, climates, aromas, and people that correspond to these and other qualities.

It is important, therefore, for the student of Ayurveda to develop the faculties of direct observation with all the senses, including the intuition. Through such observation, one becomes the Seer of one's life, making choices as needed from moment to moment—a skill analogous to a sailor using his knowledge of the winds and tides to steer a steady course. As directors of our own lives we need to know how to shift and regain balance, in both the inner and outer universe of our being.

Ayurveda: Cosmology as Physiology

The cosmology or creation theory of Ayurveda is complex as well as enlightening, with volume after volume dedicated to its exposition. In brief, the ancient Seers surmised that in the beginning there were two fundamental principles of existence, an absolute, unmanifested state of consciousness, called *Purusha*, and the principle of creativity or primal nature, called *Prakruti*. The interplay of these two principles, of Spirit and Matter, produce the physical world and the laws that govern it.

Prakruti is said to contain three *gunas*, or attributes, which are the foundation of all existence: *sattva*, the principle of light, intelligence, perception, and harmony; *rajas*, the principle of energy, activity, and turbulence; and *tamas*, the principle of inertia, darkness, dullness, and resistance.

Sattva, as subjective consciousness, is responsible for our perceptions, as well as for the clarity of those perceptions. In nature, sattva's balancing energy creates the seasons and other life rhythms. In the mind, sattva creates peace, virtue, and love. It also brings about the awakening of the soul and the five senses, opening us up to the experience of the physical universe.

Rajas is manifested as action and movement. In nature, we see the principle of rajas in various activities, from the wind blowing, to cars moving, to energy flowing. In the mind, rajas creates agitation, aggression, competition, and turbulence. From rajas are created the five motor organs of action, "the mouth for speech, the hands for grasping, the feet for moving, the genitals for emission, the anus for excretion."

Tamas gives to the world a certain steadiness and solidity—the inertia of rock, the stability of mountains—and in the body creates deep sleep or unconsciousness. Tamas in the mind, however, is responsible for periods of mental confusion and depression. From tamas come the five elements: space (sometimes called "ether"), air, fire, water, and earth.

Although all three attributes are needed to create the physical world, in the mind it is the cultivation of sattva that enables a person to feel the peace, honesty, and truth of his or her existence. Ayurveda, by emphasizing the sattvic lifestyle, moves the other gunas into a more harmonized state. The balance of the three gunas is called "pure sattva." Through healthy diet, peaceful lifestyle choices, love, faith, nonviolence, and other sattvic attributes, one experiences inner peace.

The Five Elements

All things in the physical world, including our bodies, are made up of five elements:

Space, often translated as "ether," represents the expansion of consciousness. The "space" in our mind is the place where we experience love and compassion. Similarly, each of the body's cells contains "space"; without it, there would be no communication between cells.

Air represents the gaseous form of matter, the movement of consciousness, as well as the nerve and sensory impulses. Our breathing, sense of touch and movement are all governed by the air principle, as is the movement of our thoughts and ideas.

Fire represents the radiant form of matter. Air creates movement and friction, which in turn creates heat, or "fire." In the body, "fire" is responsible for digestion, absorption and assimilation. In the mind, it accounts for our ability to understand, comprehend and realize. We perceive the world around us because of the "fire" in our eyes, which digests the contents of vision. We can see the soul of a person by the light and fire in his or her eyes.

Water represents the liquid form of matter, and the "liquefaction" of consciousness. In the body, the water principle exists as plasma, saliva, mucus, sweat, urine, cerebro-spinal fluid, and other moist components. In the mind, it exists as feelings of compassion, faith, love, and devotion.

Earth represents the solid form of matter, as well as the more crystallized manifestations of consciousness. According to Ayurveda, the molecules of the physical world are solidified consciousness. In the body, all the solid structures—bones, cartilage, teeth, nails, hair, and skin—are composed of the earth element. In the mind, the earth element is responsible for our feelings of groundedness and solidity.

Tri-dosha—The Three Constitutions

According to Ayurveda, there are three primary life forces, or biological humors, in the body, called "doshas." The doshas bind the five elements down into living flesh. These are called in Sanskrit *vata*, *pitta*, and *kapha*. They are the active and mobile elements that determine the life processes of growth and decay. Dosha literally means "that which darkens, spoils, or causes things to decay," for when out of balance they are the causative forces in the disease process.

Vata: the Air/Space Constitution

Associated with the elements of air and space, vata means "wind" or "that which moves things," and represents the force that governs biological activity. It is the prime impetus of the nervous system, controlling both sensory and mental balance, mental adaptability, and understanding. It is the basic life force (*prana*), and is enhanced by the consumption of pure, whole foods, the breathing of clean air, and by our connection with the Divine within, the deepest energizing force for the entire body.

Physiologically, vata governs:
- breathing
- inhalation/exhalation
- blinking of the eyelids
- movements in the muscles and tissues
- pulsations of the heart

- all contractions and expansions within the body
- movements and signals in the nerve cells
- digestion
- elimination/urine/menstruation/birthing

Mentally and emotionally, vata governs:
- mental power and movement coordination
- adaptability
- inspirations
- spiritual aspirations
- nervousness
- fear
- anxiety

Vata's main locations are:
- colon
- hips
- thighs
- ears
- bones
- organ of touch (skin)
- nerve tissues

In the mind, vata represents flexibility, ability to communicate, and creative resources. When aggravated, it can also manifest as insecurities, fears, and anxieties. In our bodies, vata is the movement of the nervous system, accumulating in the large intestines as gas, in the pelvic cavity as pains and aches, in the bones as arthritis, in the skin as neuralgia, in the ears as ringing, and in the hips and thighs as sciatic pain. If the body develops an excess of vata (air qualities), these are the first areas in which it will accumulate. When not deranged or out of balance, vata functions as nervous and mental force throughout the body, and is centered in the brain and the nervous system in general.

Vata is the vital motivating force behind the other two humors, which are in themselves incapable of movement.

The qualities of vata (air) are:
- light
- cold
- rough
- dry
- clear
- agitated
- subtle
- hard
- dispersing
- mobile

Vata rules:
- movement
- catabolism (breaking down of substances in the body)
- astringent taste (has a drying quality)
- old age (people tend to be drier and colder as they age)
- dawn and dusk (changing, transitional times)
- fall season (cold, dry, windy season)

Vata Disorders:
- emaciation
- loss of warmth
- tremors
- bloating
- constipation
- insomnia
- sensory disorientation
- incoherent speech
- dizziness
- confusion

- depression
- anxiety, nervousness
- migrating pain
- arthritis

Vata Characteristics

Just as the wind blows gently or forcefully in different directions, so the vata individual will manifest irregularity in his or her structure.

Build: Vata may be very tall (taller than the average in his or her family) or very short, with a tendency to be slender or rangy, a thin body frame, and narrow shoulders or hips. The arms may be unusually short or long. Vata people may have light, small bones, with prominent or protruding joints that tend to make cracking noises. Deviated nasal septum, bowlegs and knock-knees are also due to vata.

Weight: Vata is dry, creating a tendency to leanness in the predominantly vata constitution. Vata people may find it hard or impossible to gain weight, while some may overeat poor-quality foods and become fat; others may gain and lose weight erratically. Again, this is all part of vata's overall irregularity.

Complexion and Skin Characteristics: Vatas tend to be dark (relative to others of their race) and to tan deeply without burning. They are by nature cold, and therefore enjoy warm weather and sunlight.

Due to their high energy output, vata people tend to have dry skin that uses up lubricating dermal oils. However, due to vata's variability some areas of the skin may be dry while others are oily. Vata people may develop psoriasis, dry eczema, corns, calluses or chapped lips. They may show wrinkles at a young age. Because they do not store up enough energy to maintain body warmth, they feel cold to the touch. Many suffer from poor circulation, with the skin showing a grayish tinge.

Hair: Hair is closely related to prana, the life force of the body. Vata hair may vary from dry to oily in different areas of the head. It is often coarse in texture, dull and lusterless, and prone to dandruff or split ends.

Nails: Vata people have hard, rough, brittle nails that may differ in size, with marked ridges or depressions. Many times the fingers will be very cold, and bluish or grayish in color. Nail-biting is a vata attribute.

Eyes: Vata eyes may be grey, violet, slate blue, or dark chocolate. Different color eyes are also a vata characteristic. Vata eyes may be dry and scratchy, with the sclera (white part of the eye) having a grayish or bluish tinge, or dull and lusterless.

Mouth: Vata people may have crooked or uneven teeth with a mouth too large or small in proportion to the rest of the face. The teeth will tend to be brittle and oversensitive, with gums that recede early. If there is a coating on the tongue it will be thin, adherent, and grayish or pink-gray in color.

Appetite: The vata appetite is variable, with excess hunger one day and no appetite the next. If vata people do not eat regularly, they may become dizzy and weak. They do not do well with fasts, as their bodies do not store enough fat and energy to carry them through a period of food deprivation. Although vatas seem to be the people who fast the most—for purposes of cleansing, so that they can realize their spiritual aspirations more clearly—fasting may work against them, provoking the negative effects of vata.

Vatas must have breakfast; otherwise they will become anxious and tired as their blood-sugar levels drop. They may rely on caffeine to wake them up and get them going, but this will rob them of energy later in the day and will eventually exhaust them altogether by drying out their glands. (Vata tiredness is often due to adrenal exhaustion.)

Digestion/Evacuation: Vata people are usually lifelong sufferers from constipation, with frequent gas and bloating, and a tendency to hard, dark-colored stools. They respond only to strong laxatives, such as cascara sagrada and castor oil. Vatas must be reminded that good eating habits are essential for easy digestion and smooth bowel movement.

Menstruation: Vata women have irregular cycles, and may miss periods if they exercise too much or if they lose too much weight. The flow is scanty, with clots due to vata dryness. Severe cramping and constipation, lasting for hours or days, may occur before bleeding begins.

Climate: Vatas feel generally cold and dry, and enjoy warm and humid climates. They tend to be weaker during the winter and must learn to bundle up if they go out in the cold. Warming tonic herbs, such as dong quai and codonopsis, may be helpful for vatas during the winter months.

Sex: Although vata types may spend much time thinking intensely about sex, their sexual appetites vary. Vata men may experience premature ejaculation. Fertility may be lower than average in the vata person.

Physical Activity: Vata types are active and restless, with low stamina. They may drive themselves to exhaustion with overactivity and excess nervous energy. Aerobics and other rigorous exercise tire them out. Gentle, slow exercises or yoga are more appropriate.

Pulse: The vata pulse is thin, fast and said to "slither like a cobra."

Sleep: Again, the variability of vatas plays a part in their sleep patterns. They may toss and turn, or wake up frequently during the night.

Emotions: Vata people in balance may be enthusiastic, idealistic, and visionary. However, a vata who has not practiced inner quiet and a peaceful lifestyle will experience fear or anxiety when confronted with difficult situations in life.

Speech/Mind: Vatas may talk very fast and breathlessly. They have original minds, and are not afraid of new ideas or sudden inspirations. They like to communicate and put ideas together. On the other hand, they may have a hard time putting ideas into action. If undisciplined, they can be spacy and chaotic.

The Vata, and Vata-Pacifying, Lifestyles

Joe wakes up in the morning and quickly gets dressed for work. He drinks a cup of coffee, which stimulates the nervous system, and grabs a quick bite at a fast-food restaurant, which he eats while driving 65 mph through the desert outside Santa Fe—high, dry, cold, clear, windy, rough, agitated, energetic vata country. Joe rushes into work and begins to talk for hours on the phone. When lunchtime comes, he eats a salad and soft drink at his desk.

Let's see if we can pick out some of the vata elements in this story.

• First, the coffee which overstimulates the nervous system, resulting in agitation (vata), excess mobility (vata) and dryness (vata). Also, coffee is bitter and astringent (both vata qualities).

• Eating while driving is vata behavior.

- Fast foods, overcooked and lacking in nourishment, are vata.
- The salad, which is cold, light and mobile, moves through us quickly without providing deep, "building" nourishment.
- The carbonated drink, which has many gas bubbles and is cold, will increase vata qualities of lightness and coldness, and induce flatulence or burping.
- Talking all day and eating at one's desk create agitation, anxiety, indigestion, lack of inner peace, pains, tremors, twitching, and, eventually, general nervous exhaustion.

Certain lifestyle modifications will help to keep vata in balance:

Joe wakes up in the morning with a feeling of gratefulness for the day ahead. He gets out of bed and does a few gentle stretches and some deep breathing. Before his shower, he applies sesame oil to his body and allows it to stay on for a few minutes while he boils some water for spicy herbal tea and oatmeal. He takes a warm shower and puts on some comfortable natural-fiber clothing. Just before eating, he gives thanks for the nourishment and proceeds to eat his breakfast with quiet music in the background. He drives at a reasonable speed to work while listening to still more relaxing music. When lunchtime comes, Joe makes sure to get away from his desk. He orders warm vegetable soup with whole-grain bread.

This type of routine is decidedly sattvic, inducing inner peace. It will keep Joe's vata nature from getting out of hand. He feels physically better, retaining access to vata inspiration and mental acuity. Such lifestyle choices decrease the tendency to dispersion, fear, anxiety, and nervousness.

It should be mentioned that the sesame oil is warming and nourishing to the nerves, and will alleviate vata's dryness, agitation, and coldness. The warm, cooked foods are deeply nourishing and will counteract the attributes of cold, light, dryness, roughness, and hardness. In order to keep vata in its place, we must engage in practices that contrast with vata attributes: calm versus agitated, warm versus cold, soft versus hard, and so forth.

The vata person is blessed with a flexible, quick mind. There is never a lack of creative ideas and resources. Because vata is associated with motion, vata people like to be "on the move" physically, mentally, and emotionally. However, should all this nervous energy get out of hand, the vata individual may become ill with nervous exhaustion, constipation, tremors, arthritis, and so forth. The purpose of any vata-pacifying lifestyle and diet is to help regulate this motion, so that the person may continue to be inspired, but not burn out. (We will discuss vata-pacifying foods and choices in the next chapter.)

I have noticed in my practice that the biggest difficulty in working with vata people is that they often have poor follow-through with the routine suggested by the practitioner-herbalist. They get very excited about the information, but may not be grounded enough to keep the program going.

Pitta: the Fire/Water Constitution

Pitta—the biological fire humor, or "bile," means "that which digests things" or "that which heats, cooks, or transforms." It is the fire that digests the food we eat and gives our bodies warmth. Our internal fires determine our capacity to perceive reality and our power to digest life experiences.

The person with pitta predominant in her constitution is blessed with great willpower and initiative, the capacity to laugh at her troubles, great determination to reach her goals, a penetrating mind, and, usually, good "fires" for digestion.

Pitta is our enthusiasm for life, our joy and laughter. It finds negative expression in burning sensations in the body and mind, in a drive toward unhealthy competition and anger, and in the need to control.

Physiologically, pitta governs:
- hunger
- thirst
- luster
- complexion
- digestion
- body heat

Mentally and emotionally, pitta governs:
- laughter
- joy
- willpower
- enthusiasm
- anger
- competition
- judgment
- criticalness
- mental perception
- discriminating awareness
- penetrating thought
- courage

Pitta's main locations are:
- small intestine
- stomach (as digestive acids)
- blood
- eyes
- sweat
- sebaceous glands (glands that supply oil for the hair and skin)

Pitta is our inner digestive fire, acids, and bile, all of which help to combust food, providing energy and warmth. It is also the light and heat of the body and the mind.

The qualities of pitta (fire) are:
- hot
- sharp
- flowing
- light
- liquid
- oily
- smooth
- aggressive
- penetrating

Pitta rules:
- transformation
- adulthood
- metabolism (transformation of a substance)
- sour or pungent (spicy) tastes
- noon and midnight
- late spring and summer

Pitta Disorders:
- yellow stool, urine, eyes, and skin
- excess hunger
- excess thirst
- burning sensations in the body
- difficult, restless sleep
- heat, fever, inflammation
- herpes
- burning eczema and rashes
- sties ("red eye")
- liver problems
- burning, bleeding ulcers

Pitta Characteristics

Build: "Balanced" and "proportional" are the operative words for pitta. Medium-length fingers and toes, medium-width shoulders and hips, proportional frame and height.

Weight: Pittas have average weight for their height, with minor fluctuations. Fat is deposited evenly throughout the body.

Complexion: Pitta skin may be pale, pink, or copper in hue, and warm to the touch. It will tend to be delicate, irritable, and prone to rashes, pimples, and inflammations. It may have freckles, black, brown, or red moles, may sunburn easily or suffer from sun allergy, and may wrinkle early. Body hair may be light-hued and fine-textured. The lips may be deep red, showing ample blood beneath the skin. Pitta people may blush easily or turn red when angry. They may perspire very easily, even in cold weather. They may feel hot most of the time, no matter the season.

Hair: Red hair is an indication of substantial pitta in one's basic constitution. Pitta people may have light hair, or their hair may turn grey or white at an early age. Early baldness is also a pitta indicator, since it indicates high levels of testosterone, a hot, pitta-type hormone. The hair is thin, fine, or delicate, and usually quite straight. It may be oily as well.

Nails: Pitta nails are soft, strong, rubbery and well-formed. They may be very pink in color, with a coppery tinge due to a profusion of warm blood right under the skin.

Eyes: Pitta eyes are medium in size, and may be light in color. Pitta eyes may also be hazel, green, or light blue, and may be tinged with red. The eyes look as though they are burning with an intense fire, and radiate high levels of energy. The sclera (white of the eyes) may have a reddish tinge and become fiery red when irritated.

Mouth: Pittas have medium-sized teeth, prone to cavities and bleeding gums. The tongue coating may be yellow, orange, or red. The tongue itself may be irritated or bleed. Pitta-predominant people often get canker sores and experience a sour or metallic taste in the mornings.

Appetite: Pittas usually have good appetites and enjoy eating. They hate to miss meals and will grow irritable if they fail to eat when they are hungry. They do not like to fast, and if they do, may become quite agitated. In general, they like to consume and absorb new energy.

If pittas skip breakfast they will be ravenous by noon. However, if they are focused on a goal, they may skip a meal and remember later that they haven't eaten all day.

Digestion/Evacuation: Pittas are usually not constipated, enjoying frequent bowel movements. Many times the stool has a yellowish tinge and is well-formed, although it may also be loose, hot, and burning. Intense yellow or orange stool may indicate great pitta intensity (or too much salsa and chips). If a pitta person does suffer from occasional constipation, milk, figs, raisins, or dates may serve as a laxative.

Menstruation: Pittas have regular cycles, but may bleed longer and heavier than others due to their innate heat. The blood is bright red. Pitta women may have loose stools during or just before their periods. They may also experience heat and sweating before menstruation. If they have cramps, these are of medium strength.

Climate: Pittas find hot climates intolerable.

Sex: Pittas have ample sex drives and, when aroused, tend to pursue their goals. They can be quite romantic, although when thwarted they may grow angry and flare up. They are average in fertility.

Physical Activity: Pittas can endure much vigorous exercise as long as they do not grow overheated.

Pulse: The pitta pulse is full, regular, and strong, with medium speed and rhythm. In pure pitta, it is said to "jump like a frog."

Sleep: Pittas tend to go to sleep easily and sleep lightly, but if they are awakened during the night, have no trouble going to sleep again.

Emotions: Pittas can be "intense." Sometimes, because of the heat in their body, they may react with immediate anger to challenging situations. (This may or may not manifest outwardly.) However, many pittas I know are able to laugh at adversity and enjoy challenges.

Speech/Mind: Pittas are usually precise and direct in what they say. They have an acute intelligence and tend to be impatient with anyone whose intelligence is not equal to theirs. They often want to dominate. They are methodical and efficient, and love steering ideas into practical applications.

The Pitta, and Pitta-Pacifying, Lifestyles

Jill lives in East Texas, where the summers are hot and humid, the sun so bright she has to squint her eyes to see. Jill decides to go out for a short jog, then have a bite to eat. She puts on a red running suit, laces up her sneakers and jogs to town. At the local cantina, she indulges herself with salsa and chips, followed by a spicy meat-and-bean burrito smothered in hot sauce. After her feast, she feels a little irritated about the service that she received in the restaurant and begins to tell the manager everything that is wrong with the waiter. She leaves the restaurant feeling flushed, hot and bothered.

First of all, East Texas is a predominantly pitta environment—bright, humid, aggressively hot. The red running suit is likewise hot and aggressive in nature, and jogging is a very overheating type of exercise, especially in the summer. The food too is hot, sharp, penetrating, oily—basically pitta in nature. The emotions of rash judgment and keen irritation are signs that Jill's pitta is elevated.

Now let's look at a pitta-pacifying scenario:

Jill looks outside and sees that it is another hot, sweltering day. She decides to wear a cool, light blue summer dress and anoint herself with sandalwood oil. She drives to town in her air-conditioned car, to a salad bar that has a lovely garden atmosphere with a small waterfall and pond. She orders a light meal with peppermint tea.

All the choices Jill has made are pitta-pacifying and, for her, quite sattvic, increasing coolness, calmness, and peacefulness.

I have noticed in my practice that the pitta people may want to control the Ayurvedic session. They may be contentious or aggressive, questioning the practitioner's credentials and status. It is best not to debate or argue with pittas. Try to gain their trust through discussion and presentation of facts. Once they know what they need to do, they will begin to implement the program—and may even do it to excess. (I have known pittas to carry their program with them on laminated cards so that they can follow it precisely.)

Pitta-predominant people—classic Type A's—have a tendency to do too much and burn themselves out. Chronic fatigue and liver ailments are not uncommon in the pitta person.

Kapha: the Water/Earth Constitution

Kapha, the biological force of water/earth, means both "phlegm" and "that which holds things together." It is the physical and emotional "home" in which we reside, providing the substance and support for our body, giving bulk to our tissues. Emotionally, kapha is the love and support we receive in life, governing feelings of compassion, devotion, modesty, patience, and forgiveness. Negatively expressed, kapha is greed, attachment, and self-pity.

Kapha helps to ground and control the active and consuming natures of vata and pitta. It exerts a conserving, consolidating, stabilizing, restraining force over the body and mind. Vata and pitta will squander their energy without kapha to hold them down. The subtle essence of all the kapha, or water, in the body is called *ojas*. Ojas is the prime energy reserve in the body and is the vitality of the immune system. If there is an excess loss of kapha due to stress, improper eating, and illness, we will suffer from a compromised immune system and will lack both physical and emotional support.

Physiologically, kapha governs:
- form and solidity
- storing of energy
- stability
- lubrication
- holding together of the joints
- body fluids
- the sense of taste

Mentally and emotionally, kapha governs:
- patience
- forgiveness
- compassion
- love
- deep sense of satisfaction
- sense of being grounded and belonging
- attachment
- greed
- mental inertia
- dullness

Kapha's main locations are:
- stomach
- chest
- throat
- head
- pancreas
- sides
- lymph
- fat
- nose
- tongue

Its primary site is the stomach.

The qualities of kapha (water/earth) are:
- heavy
- slow
- liquid
- dense
- dull
- cold
- thick
- soft

- sticky
- cloudy
- oily
- damp

Kapha rules:
- constructing of form
- anabolism (building up of substance)
- sweet and salty tastes
- the childhood years
- morning and evening
- winter and late spring

Kapha Disorders:
- depression of digestive "fire"
- nausea after eating
- lethargy
- heaviness
- paleness
- chills
- looseness of the limbs
- cough
- difficult breathing
- mucous conditions
- excessive sleeping
- accumulation of fat in the body
- congestion of the lymphatic system

Kapha in the chest or lungs produces moisture, as it does in the throat, head, sinuses, and nasal passages. In the mouth and tongue, kapha produces saliva. (The tongue is the organ of taste, the sensory quality that is said to belong to the water element.) Kapha creates fat tissue, which stores water. It is also held along the sides of the abdominal cavity, in the form of peritoneal fluid. An excessive amount of kapha will produce an overabundance of mucus and, therefore, congestion.

Kapha Characteristics

Build: Kapha people are the bulkiest of the three different constitutions, with medium to broad frames, heavy bone structure and wide shoulders and/or hips. They store energy, which encourages massiveness. Kaphas are well-lubricated and normally experience none of the problems associated with dryness. Many kaphas have fingers that are squarish and short.

Weight: Kaphas can maintain moderate weight with regular exercise, but usually do not like to exert themselves. They gain weight easily, especially around the mid-torso and the hips, and they lose weight slowly.

Complexion: Kaphas tan evenly and enjoy the sun. The skin may be cool, but not cold, to the touch. (They do not suffer from cold hands and feet to the extent that vatas do.) Many times kaphas have very beautiful skin—smooth and soft, slightly oily, with a moderate amount of body hair and very few moles. They do not have a propensity to skin disorders, but may experience stagnation of the lymphatic system due to blockages of energy. Kaphas sweat moderately, at about the same intensity in all climates.

Hair: Kaphas usually have brown or black, thick, slightly wavy hair, sometimes bordering on coarse. Oily hair may be a problem, but the hair luster is good.

Nails: Kapha nails are strong, large, and symmetrical, with very little variation.

Eyes: Kapha eyes tend to be large, liquid, calm, cool, and stable. Some people say that Kaphas have the "eyes of a deer."

Mouth: Kaphas often have large and even teeth. If there is a coating on the tongue it may be thick, white, or off-white, with a curdled look. The taste in the mouth may be sickly sweet.

Appetite: Kaphas have a stable and moderate desire for food, although they may be prone to emotional eating. Fasting is relatively easy on them due to their ability to store energy, but it rarely occurs to them to fast. Kaphas tend not to be hungry upon awakening. They may feel hungry around 10 or 11 a.m. for a light breakfast—maybe some spicy tea and a piece of fruit—but are just as likely to skip breakfast entirely. They may want coffee to stimulate them in the a.m. Two meals per day is usually sufficient for a kapha.

Digestion/Evacuation: Kaphas have regular bowel movements, with well-formed, rarely hard stools. (When constipated, they respond to medium-strength laxatives.) Kapha people may be prone to yeast conditions due to the dampness in their system, causing digestive problems. Also, they may feel heavy and lethargic after eating, due to overall slow metabolism and sluggish digestion.

Menstruation: Kaphas may have effortless, regular periods with an average quantity of blood, light in color. Cramps are usually mild and dull. Kaphas may be prone to water retention and edema, however.

Climate: Due to their stability, Kaphas are generally not disturbed by extremes of climate. They may prefer warm weather, but not humid. Cold, damp climates may be aggravating to kaphas and their physical complaints.

Sex: Kaphas have a steady desire for sex and enjoy it. They are slow to arouse, but once aroused can remain that way for a long time. Fertility is unusually high.

Physical Activity: Kaphas can endure vigorous exercise, but may not be interested in this kind of energy expenditure. When they do exercise it makes them feel strong and healthy.

Pulse: A kapha pulse is said to beat smoothly, "like a swan." It is full, slow, rhythmic, and the artery may feel cool and rubbery. Sometimes, however, a kapha pulse is hard to find due to the firmness of the flesh at the wrist area.

Sleep: Kaphas drop off quickly, sleep heavily, and wake up rested and alert. They like to oversleep to store up energy.

Emotions: Kaphas like to avoid confrontations due to their innate sweetness, which may lead to complacency. They do not like change and are stressed by unpredictable situations. They are predominantly calm, quiet, steady, and serious, and enjoy home and family. Kapha in excess may be too passive, attached, possessive, and greedy. Once they get moving and are committed to a course of action, kaphas will generally see it through.

Speech/Mind: Kaphas may speak slowly and cautiously, without volunteering much—information must be pulled out of them. They will initiate a conversation only if they have something to say. The kapha voice may be quite melodious.

The Kapha, and Kapha-Pacifying, Lifestyles

On a cold, damp morning in Seattle, Pat opens her eyes, curls up in the down comforter and tries to catch a few more minutes of sleep. After a while, she lazily gets out of her waterbed and gets ready for work. She puts on some very sweet-smelling rose perfume and a pink, fluffy outfit. At work, the do-nut man comes around 10 a.m.—Pat purchases three donuts and a carton of cold milk. Her job at the bank keeps her sitting most of the day. At lunch, Pat orders fried chicken, french fries, cold Diet Coke, and frozen yogurt. When she goes home at night, she turns on the TV and eats nachos with extra cheese, followed by more frozen yogurt.

Cold, damp, low-elevation climates—such as that of Seattle—are kapha in nature. Sleepiness and inertia are kapha attributes. The donuts contain the sweet taste that increases kapha. The same applies to the rose perfume and pink garments; both color and aroma are sweet in nature. The sedentary job reinforces kapha's heavy, slow, thick, static, soft, dull nature. Fried chicken, french fries, cheese, frozen yogurt, and cold drinks increase the physical qualities of heaviness, slowness, coldness, oiliness, denseness, thickness, stickiness, and dullness, and will also increase mental dullness, emotional fixations, overindulgence, and greed. Waterbeds are too soft—and watery—for kapha persons.

Let us take a look at a kapha-pacifying story for Pat:

It is a cold, damp day in Seattle, so Pat keeps the house warm and dry. She sleeps on a relatively hard bed—comfortable, but not too soft or sumptuous. When she wakes up she gets out of bed immediately and does some deep-breathing and mild aerobics for a minute or two, to get the blood flowing. Before her shower, she uses a loofa sponge to dry-brush her body in order to stimulate the lymphatic system. For breakfast, she has some stewed fruit and a spicy tea. She forgoes

snacks at work and has a nourishing lunch of steamed veg-
etables, grains and salad, followed by a spicy warm drink
and a walk before returning to work. At night she has a
light meal and does not eat anything else until morning.

Kapha people have great strength and endurance. They also have faith in life, and in those close to them. They can provide the stable, nurturing, grounded energy that is so rare—and so needed—these days.

I have noticed in my practice that kapha people must be treated with firmness, and aggressively enough to move them out of their complacency. You must lovingly tell them what will happen if they do not do something to overcome their inertia. They need to be motivated and put on a strict, rigorous regimen.

Prakruti/Vikruti:
Constitutional Amendments

Within each of us is a place of balance and equilibrium, our basic nature or constitution, which Ayurveda calls *prakruti*. Prakruti is the combination of the three doshas (vata, pitta and kapha) that we received at conception, and so refers to the individual's inherent, inborn tendencies or "nature." Prakruti never changes during our lifetime. Prakruti influences activity as well as consciousness, and determines how our body-mind will respond to stress.

We also have our current state, our situation "at the moment." This is called *vikruti*. When a person is more or less free of discomfort, we can assume that his or her prakruti (inherent constitution) and vikruti (current condition) are somewhat in balance. Unfortunately, diet, lifestyle, age, emotions, environment, and so forth have a way of knocking one's constitution out of balance.

Some Ayurvedic practitioners have found it useful to attach a numerical value to the levels of vata (V), pitta (P) and kapha (K) that constitute an individual's prakruti. For the purposes of this pocket guide, the highest value level will be 4, the lowest 1.

My prakruti, for example, is:

V1, P3, K2

In other words, my prakruti is predominantly pitta, with lesser or secondary amounts of vata and kapha.

Now let's say I am lecturing, traveling extensively and therefore keeping irregular hours. Because of this, I may begin to suffer from insomnia, dry sensations in the body, gas and constipation. Because of lifestyle choices, a rough measurement of my current constitution (vikruti) shows elevated vata. I must now take remedial measures to bring vata down to its usual place of V1.

Your prakruti is the place where your health is. We are not trying to have vata, pitta, and kapha in equal proportions, which would contradict our basic natures. We are trying to honor that with which we were born, our place of balance.

Let me give another example. Again, my prakruti is:

V1, P3, K2

On a hot summer day, I decide to have a big Italian meal with lots of garlic and tomato sauce. Later that night, I begin to feel burning sensations in the intestines. My stool is very loose and burns as well. There is a slight rash on my face, and I generally feel irritated.

The foods that I ate are pitta- or fire-provoking; therefore my current situation, or vikruti, shows elevated pitta that needs to be brought down to its usual place of P3. Only then will I begin to feel well. I should take some pitta-pacifying herbs and make the appropriate lifestyle choices to bring pitta down to its proper level. (Very often a person's predominant dosha is the one that becomes unbalanced most easily.)

Because many Western treatments and medicines work with symptoms, but fail to take into account our true natures, they may throw us even more out of balance. Trying to handle a situation with more and more complicated therapies may further remove us from the simplicity and innocence of nature and our deeper selves. Health is our natural state. The aim in Ayurveda is to restore our basic nature (prakruti) and help us to live in harmony with it.

Finding Out Your Basic Constitution (Prakruti) and Current Conditions (Vikruti)

When taking the following test, keep in mind that we are trying to determine prakruti. Base your choices on what has been most constant in your life over a considerable time period. A separate test for vikruti follows.

Constitutional (Prakruti) Evaluation

Things to remember when taking the test:

1. Certain fixed attributes—such as body frame, weight, shape of arms and legs, and complexion—plus the state of metabolism and digestion give us a good indicator of your prakruti.

2. Lifelong habits and proclivities are also good indicators.

3. If you feel that two or three statements in some of the categories fit you, mark them all down. Mark on each line that applies to you the letter V, P, or K, then count up the total number of each letter.

4. If you do not have a clear picture of yourself in some areas, have a friend help you clarify where you stand in relation to some of the questions.

1. Body Structure:

____ Vata—taller or shorter than average; thin, wiry build

__P__ Pitta—medium height; moderately developed physique

____ Kapha—stout, stocky, well-developed physique; may be tall but solidly built

2. Weight:
____ Vata—low weight, or variable weight gain and loss; prominent veins and bones
_P_ Pitta—moderate weight; good muscle tone
____ Kapha—heavy, firm; may be obese

3. Complexion: (Take into consideration racial background):
____ Vata—dull, brown or grayish hue; dark overall
_P_ Pitta—red hue; ruddy, flushed, glowing
____ Kapha—white, pale; not too red or flushed

4. Skin Texture and Temperature:
____ Vata—thin, dry, cold, cracked, rough; may have prominent veins
_P_ Pitta—warm, moist, pink; may have moles, freckles, acne
____ Kapha—white, thick-skinned, cool, soggy, soft, smooth, oily

5. Hair:
____ Vata—dry, coarse, scanty
____ Pitta—fine, soft; may gray early; tendency to baldness
_K_ Kapha—oily, thick; wavy, lustrous, abundant

6. Eyes:
____ Vata—small, dry, dull, unsteady; may blink a lot; erratic eye movement
_P_ Pitta—medium size; may have red sclera (whites) or inflamed eyes; the eyes have a "piercing" quality and may be sensitive to light
____ Kapha—wide, prominent; white sclera

7. Face:
____ Vata—long, thin, small; may wrinkle early
__P__ Pitta—sharp features; moderate size
____ Kapha—round, large; soft contours

8. Shoulders:
__P__ Vata—thin, small, hunched; may have a caved-in chest
____ Pitta—medium size
____ Kapha—broad, well-developed

9. Arms:
____ Vata—may be too long or short for body; underdeveloped, may be bony
__P__ Pitta—medium arms with moderate build
____ Kapha—thick, round, well-developed

10. Joints:
____ Vata—dry, with popping or cracking sounds
__P__ Pitta—medium, soft, loose; may experience inflammation
____ Kapha—thick joints

11. Legs:
____ Vata—thin, often excessively long or short; bony knees
__P__ Pitta—medium-sized legs, medium strength
____ Kapha—large, stocky

12. Nails:
____ Vata—thin, brittle, dry, cracked; possibly bitten
__P__ Pitta—soft, pink, well-formed
____ Kapha—smooth, firm, large, white

13. Urine:
__✓__ Vata—scanty, colorless
____ Pitta—profuse, dark yellow or light brown

_____ Kapha—may be milky white in color

14. Stools:
_✓_ Vata—dry, hard, difficult evacuation accompanied by gas; tendency to constipation and irregularity
_____ Pitta—loose, abundant amount; sometimes yellowish in color
_____ Kapha—moderate amount, solid, well-formed; may have mucus in stool

15. Appetite:
_✓_ Vata—erratic, i.e., fine one day followed the next by gas and poor digestion; or hungry one day, not so the next
_____ Pitta—strong appetite; will become irritated if he or she does not eat on time
_____ Kapha—consistent appetite, slow metabolism; may eat to cope with negative emotions

16. Circulation:
_____ Vata—poor, variable; cold hands, cold feet, cold body
_____ Pitta—good circulation; warm
_K_ Kapha—slow circulation; cool hands, warm body

17. Activity:
_P_ Vata—fast, changeable, erratic; hyperactive
_____ Pitta—motivated, goal-oriented, intense, competitive, aggressive
_____ Kapha—slow, deliberate, steady

18. Sensitivity:
_✓_ Vata—sensitive to wind, cold, and dryness
_P_ Pitta—sensitive to heat, fire; aggravated by too much sun
_K_ Kapha—sensitive to cold, damp, foggy areas; likes the sun

19. Disease Tendency:

___ Vata—nervous-system diseases, arthritis, migrating aches and pains, intestinal disorders, gas, mental/emotional disorders

___ Pitta—fevers, infections, inflammations, ulcers, colitis, blood diseases, rashes, red itching skin diseases, heat

___ Kapha—mucus diseases, respiratory problems, water retention, blockages, depression

20. Resistance:

___ Vata—variable resistance; may have weak immune system

___ Pitta—medium resistance; prone to infections, heat, inflammatory conditions

___ Kapha—high resistance; generally strong immunity

21. Medications:

___ Vata—may experience rapid, unexpected reactions to medication; low doses

___ Pitta—medium reactions; medium doses

___ Kapha—slow reactions; high doses

22. Voice:

___ Vata—may be deep, weak, grating due to lack of moisture

___ Pitta—Sharp, penetrating; may be high-pitched

___ Kapha—soothing quality, deep, good tone

23. Speech:

___ Vata—quick, talkative, erratic

___ Pitta—moderate, convincing, intense, argumentative, forceful

___ Kapha—quiet, deliberate, slow

24. Sleep:

___✓___ Vata—light sleeper; may suffer from insomnia, wakes up at night and stays up worrying

_____ Pitta—moderate sleeper; goes back to sleep easily

_____ Kapha—heavy sleeper; sleeps deeply, but may be groggy upon awakening

25. Pulse:

_____ Vata—the pulse will be fast, feeble, "slithery," with 80–100 beats per minute

___P___ Pita—the pulse will feel "like a frog jumping," excited and prominent, with a moderate rate of 60–75 beats per minute

_____ Kapha—the pulse will be strong, regular, broad, steady, and slow, 60–70 beats per minute, and may be hard to find due to fat and thick tissue at the wrist area

Count the number of times you selected V, P, and K, and place the totals in the appropriate boxes below.

Next, determine from the scale below the relative strength for each dosha. For example if your total for vata was 7, then the vata part of your prakruti will be 2. If the total for the pitta is 16, your pitta part will be 3. If your kapha total is 2, your kapha part is 1.

Total Vata__8__   Total Pitta__16__   Total Kapha__4__

         1–6 = a designation of 1
         7–12 = a designation of 2
         13–18 = a designation of 3
         18–24 = a designation of 4

My prakruti is: V__2__ P__3__ K__1__

In all, there are seven different prakruti possibilities:
- Predominantly vata
- Predominantly pitta
- Predominantly kapha
- Equal amounts of:
  - vata/pitta
  - vata/kapha
  - pitta/kapha
  - vata/pitta/kapha

Current Condition (Vikruti) Evaluation

When you have a minor or serious imbalance, certain symptoms can be evaluated as vata, pitta, or kapha in nature. While prakruti is what we are born with, vikruti will show us what is out of balance. To determine the vikruti it is important to evaluate the dosha of the condition as it is manifesting. One easy way to do this is to list all the symptoms, then try to evaluate each one to see if it is vata, pitta, or kapha in nature. For example, if you have indigestion, try to describe to yourself the feelings associated with it, such as: "sour burps and burning sensation in the stomach and colon. I develop a rash on my face after eating." This would indicate a pitta digestive disorder. Vikruti must be dealt with until the symptoms have cleared; then we can go back to our lifestyle and diet choices for prakruti.

It should be noted that some people have been out of balance for so long that they cannot figure out what the prakruti is until some of the imbalances are taken care of. That which is manifesting *now* must be addressed first. With complicated conditions, more than one dosha may be out of balance. I have provided some suggestions as to how to handle this type of situation. It may be best to obtain the advice of an Ayurvedic consultant for more serious illnesses.

This test will give you an idea as to how to evaluate your current condition. You do not have to answer all the questions, as some of them may not apply to your situation. The number that is the highest will show you your vikruti. Follow the diet and lifestyle considerations until the situation is handled and you are feeling better. Then return to the diet for your prakruti.

You may find that your vikruti is an exacerbation of your prakruti. For example, if you have a pitta prakruti you may find that the vikruti is pitta in nature also. The most prominent dosha in our constitution is often the one that becomes aggravated. This test is geared toward evaluating the acute conditions of colds, flu, cough, and stomach distress.

1. Complexion:
____ Vata—dark, brown, sallow
____ Pitta—red, yellow, rashes
____ Kapha—white, pale

2. Mucus:
____ Vata—clear, light, very runny
____ Pitta—yellow, green, maybe some blood
____ Kapha—white to clear, heavy, "stuck"

3. Circulation:
____ Vata—coldness in the body; hard to keep warm
____ Pitta—generally hot; sometimes heat in different areas of the body
____ Kapha—generally cool; possibly cold hands and feet

4. Discharges:
____ Vata—gas, burping, popping joints
____ Pitta—bleeding, pus, inflammation, rashes
____ Kapha—salivation, excess moisture

5. Quality of Pain:
____ Vata—severe, throbbing, biting, intense, variable, migratory, intermittent
____ Pitta—medium, burning
____ Kapha—heavy, dull, constant

6. Quality of Fever:
____ Vata—moderate temperature, variable or irregular; thirst, anxiety, restlessness
____ Pitta—high temperature, burning sensation; thirst, sweating, irritability, delirium
____ Kapha—low-grade fever; dullness, heaviness; constant elevated temperature

7. Unusual Tastes in the Mouth:
____ Vata—astringent, dry
____ Pitta—bitter or pungent, increased salivation
____ Kapha—sweet or salty, profuse salivation, discharge of mucus

8. Quality of Cough:
____ Vata—dry cough with little mucus; difficulty with inhalation; feeling of constriction
____ Pitta—cough feels hot; phlegm has yellow or green color, possibly with blood mixed in
____ Kapha—heavy mucous condition with much congestion

9. Throat:
____ Vata—dry, rough; painful constriction of esophagus
____ Pitta—sore throat, inflammation, burning sensation
____ Kapha—swelling, dilation, edema, puffed-up feeling

10. Stomach/Digestion:

____ Vata—decreased secretions, irregular appetite, frequent belching or hiccup, tightness in the stomach, gas, bloating

____ Pitta—good appetite, but sour burps, burning sensation or ulceration

____ Kapha—slow digestion, sweet or mucousy burps, food "just sits there"

11. Stools:

____ Vata—constipation, painful and difficult bowel movements; dry stool, small in quantity

____ Pitta—diarrhea, i.e., watery stools; quick or uncontrollable evacuation; burning sensation, increased frequency, yellowish color

____ Kapha—solid; large amount with decreased frequency of elimination; may contain mucus; anus may itch

12. Urine:

____ Vata— colorless; scanty, difficult to discharge, increased frequency or absence of urination

____ Pitta—profuse, with burning sensation; increased frequency; yellow, turbid, brown, or red in color

____ Kapha—profuse with decreased frequency; mucus in urine, white or pale in color

13. Skin:

____ Vata—dry, scaly, rough

____ Pitta—red, inflamed, itchy

____ Kapha—swollen with excess water (edema)

14. Onset of Complaint:
____ Vata—rapid, variable, irregular
____ Pitta—medium, with fever
____ Kapha—slow, constant

15. Time of the Day When the Condition Is Most Aggravated:
____ Vata—dawn, dusk
____ Pitta—noon, midnight
____ Kapha—mid-morning, mid-evening

16. Season in Which Condition Is Aggravated:
____ Vata—fall, early winter
____ Pitta—summer, late spring
____ Kapha—late winter, early spring

17. External Aggravating Factors:
____ Vata—wind, cold, dryness
____ Pitta—heat, sun, fire, humidity
____ Kapha—dampness, cold

18. Foods That Seem to Aggravate the Situation:
____ Vata—Dry foods, beans, cold foods, raw foods, stale foods, carbonated drinks, caffeine
____ Pitta—hot and spicy food, salty foods, sour foods, meats, tomatoes, caffeine, acidy foods
____ Kapha—dairy foods, salt, sweets, cold drinks, fatty fried foods, caffeine

19. Emotions You Are Experiencing Now:
____ Vata—Fear, anxiety (perhaps with hyperventilation), insecurity, tremors, palpitations, instability, insomnia
____ Pitta—irritation, impatience, anger, frustration
____ Kapha—lethargy, sadness, apathy, dullness, sleepiness, depression

20. How Have You Been Sleeping?

_____ Vata—wake up at night and cannot go back to sleep; insomnia

_____ Pitta—go to sleep easily, but have disturbing dreams, night sweats, or fitful rest

_____ Kapha—sleep okay, but lethargic in the morning; excessively tired

Add up the totals for vata, pitta and kapha and enter these totals in the spaces below. (For this test, your number is the actual result of the addition, not—as in the first test—a range defined by the result of the addition.) Follow the pacifying diet for the dosha that is the highest or most notably out of balance relative to the prakruti (basic condition) scale.

Vata_____   Pitta_____   Kapha_____

For example: V8, P2, K3. The vata-pacifying routine would be most appropriate for now.

If two doshas are equally elevated, then follow the diet and herbs that are common to both:

• If both pitta and kapha are equally elevated, note that both of these doshas respond well to bitter herbs. However, the diet should be mild and not include any dairy, which is kapha-provoking, and the spices should not be overly hot (i.e., pitta-provoking).

• If vata and pitta are equally elevated, the diet should be mild, with sweet grains and vegetables and possibly some meat protein. The spices should be mild as well. Demulcent and sweet herbs, such as marshmallow root, may be recommended, depending on the condition (see "Dietary Recommendations" in Chapter 3).

• If vata and kapha are equally elevated, follow a mild, warming diet, since both kapha and vata are cold in nature. Have lots of warm, spicy tea, and foods that are easy to digest but nourishing, such as stews and soups. Avoid cold foods and congestive foods such as dairy.

• If you notice that the symptoms are changing, then retake the vikruti test and note the results.

• After the conditions have subsided, you may go back to the diet and lifestyle recommendations for your prakruti (basic constitution).

Humans frequently become habituated to foods that do not agree with them—or which moderate or exacerbate their own worst tendencies. Vata people often become hypoglycemic because they love to eat sugar, which provides instant satisfaction by temporarily leveling out vata's mental roller coaster. Workaholic pitta people may become habituated to meat, hot spices and salt, which inflame pittas and make them even more driven, intense, and goal-oriented. Kapha people may find themselves habituated to heavy, fatty foods, which reinforce their tendency to stagnation and dullness.

We need to invoke our creative intelligence and awareness to move us toward the things and qualities that will support our deepest, truest selves. When we begin to implement changes in our lives, they should be accomplished slowly, with great awareness. Do not try to change your whole life at once, or you will be setting yourself up for failure. Decide that you will *slowly* cut down on a certain activity or food choice. And be sure to thank yourself for all the little steps you have taken toward better health.

Ayurveda and Diet

The Six Tastes

In order to understand why certain diets and herbs are recommended for each of the doshas, it is important to understand the six tastes (*rasas*) that pervade our lives.

Sweet: The sweet taste is found in sugars and starches, and is composed of the elements earth and water. Examples of sweet foods include grains, sweet vegetables, and sweet fruits. The sweet taste builds and strengthens body tissue, soothes the mucous membranes, and allays burning sensations. Sweet foods increase the quality of kapha in the body and promote calmness, contentment and harmonization of the mind. The sweet taste helps the vata person and the pitta person because both these doshas are lacking some of the grounding, building, soothing qualities of kapha. Note, however, that if a person has a kapha condition of mucus or excess fat, the sweet taste will increase these qualities. "Empty" sweets such as cakes and cookies, made with refined sweetener and flours, are deranging to all constitutions.

Salty: The salty taste is found in table salt, rock salt, sea salt, and seaweeds. It is composed of the elements water and fire. The salty taste adds warmth and moisture to the body, thus increasing kapha dampness and pitta heat. In small amounts, the salty taste aids digestion, is sedating, and softens the body tissues—all useful therapies for the vata person. Pittas and kaphas must stay away from excess salt, which will cause them aggravation.

Pungent: The pungent taste is found in hot spices such as ginger and cayenne, and contains abundant amounts of the elements fire and air. The pungent taste is heating, drying and stimulating, increasing the rate of metabolism (by about 15 percent), counteracting cold sensations and aiding in digestion. Kaphas can use a generous amount of spices in their diets to counteract their general dampness, coolness, and stagnancy. Vatas can use some spice to warm them up, but they must use it with caution because it is also drying; they ought to use spices with foods that are liquid, warm, and oily, such as soups and stews. Pittas are usually warm enough and may have problems with burning sensations, so they do not need much spice. People who are suffering from pitta conditions, such as rashes or inflammation, should also avoid spices.

Sour: The sour taste contains the elements earth and fire, and is thirst-relieving and nourishing, dispels gas and stimulates growth of bodily tissues. The sour taste is found in fermented foods such as yogurt, miso, pickles, buttermilk, and sour fruits, as well as in acidic fruits. Sour is good for vatas as it will warm, moisten, and ground them. Kaphas should not eat much that is sour as it will make them damper, and pittas may become overheated or experience burning sensations in the stomach and intestines. It should be noted that although bananas taste sweet, they have a post-digestive sour quality and may create burning sensations or aggravate ulcers (a pitta condition).

Bitter: The bitter taste contains the elements air and space, and is found in herbs such as gentian and goldenseal, and in foods such as dandelion greens and chard. The bitter taste is cooling, drying, and detoxifying, reducing all bodily tissues, and creating lightness in the body and the mind. This taste will help kaphas, because it will lighten and dry up the bulk and the water in the system. It is also good for pittas, as it cools off the heat in their liver and other areas, as well as allaying inflammation such as fevers. A vata person or a person with a vata condition should not have very many bitters in the diet, however; they will be too dehydrating.

Astringent: The drying astringent taste, composed of the elements air and earth, stops excess discharges such as sweating and diarrhea, promotes the healing of tissues, and makes the cells of the body firmer. It is good for moist kaphas because it will squeeze them out like a sponge. It is also good for pittas because it will dry up excess acids and moisture. (Remember, the elements fire *and* water dominate the pitta constitution.) Astringent herbs are good for healing wounds as well. Foods with the astringent taste include cranberries, apples, and pomegranates. Astringent herbs include oak bark, witch hazel, and raspberry leaves.

Taste and the Three Doshas

Vata

Aggravated by:	Balanced by:
bitter	sweet
astringent	sour
excess pungent	salty

Remember, we want to pacify vata, not aggravate it.

Pitta

Aggravated by:	Balanced by:
sour	sweet
pungent	bitter
salty	astringent

Sour, salty, and pungent are too heating for pitta.

Kapha

Aggravated by:	Balanced by:
sweet	pungent
salty	bitter
sour	astringent

The sweet, salty, and sour tastes have watery, building
qualities which kapha does not need.

Complex and Pure Forms of the Six Tastes

The complex forms of the tastes are less likely to aggravate vata,
pitta, or kapha, as they require more assimilation and therefore
do not have as strong or fast-acting effects as the pure forms.

Taste	Pure Form	Complex
sweet	sugar	complex carbohydrates rice, grains
salty	table salt	seaweeds
pungent	cayenne pepper garlic	mild spices such as cardamom and fennel
sour	alcohol	sour food (buttermilk)
bitter	pure bitter (gentian)	mild bitter (dandelion and aloe vera juice)
astringent	strong tannins (oak bark)	mild astringents (red raspberry)

Agni: "Digestive Fires"

Agni, named after the Hindu god of fire, is the "biological fire" that rules digestion. Agni is:

- hot
- dry
- light
- fragrant
- subtle
- mobile
- penetrating

Agni is the creative flame of transformation behind all life, as well as the acidic substance that breaks down food and stimulates digestion. Agni is increased by hot, fragrant spices such as ginger, black pepper, and cayenne, each of which has a similar nature to agni.

Agni also maintains the body's autoimmune mechanism. Strong agni destroys microorganisms, bacteria, and toxins in the stomach, as well as in the small and large intestines. It is also the protector of the good flora in the body. Skin color, the enzyme system, and metabolism all depend on agni. When agni is functioning optimally, the breakdown, absorption, and assimilation of food will be operating efficiently.

When agni becomes impaired due to an imbalance in one's constitution, the body will not receive the nutrients it needs. Eventually this will result in a breakdown of the immune system. Food material that is not digested properly becomes a foul-smelling, sticky substance that clogs the intestines and other channels, such as the blood vessels; in Ayurvedic terminology, this is called *ama*, or undigested waste. Ama accumulates, then travels through the blood to become lodged in the weakest organs. In this way, disease conditions are manifested.

Everyone, no matter what his or her constitution, should work at keeping the digestive fires strong so as not to accumulate ama, which reduces general health and clarity of mind.

Pitta types may have high agni. If it is too high due to an excess of digestive acids, the food may go through the system too quickly, resulting in burning sensations. Vatas may have irregular agni: one day they can eat anything, the next day everything bothers them. Kaphas tend to have low agni, and therefore exhibit slow metabolism and heaviness.

Agni is improved by:
- eating the foods appropriate for your constitution (prakruti) or current condition (vikruti)
- chewing well
- eating smaller portions
- properly spicing foods
- taking a small amount of bitter herbs, such as dandelion extract or artichoke extract, before meals. (Bitter extracts may be purchased at health-food stores; take 20–40 drops 15 minutes before meals.)
- eating clean, natural, fresh foods
- eating fruit and vegetables in season

Agni is impaired by:
- overeating
- drinking cold or iced drinks, which put out the digestive fires
- drinking alcohol with meals
- eating too quickly
- eating poor food combinations
- watching TV, reading, or driving when eating
- eating when upset
- drinking coffee with or after meals
- eating denatured, stale, lifeless food
- eating microwaved foods, which had their "life force" destroyed

Dietary Recommendations

For predominantly vata, pitta, or kapha:
Follow the dietary recommendations for your prominent dosha throughout the year, making appropriate seasonal adjustments when necessary.

For vata-pitta:
Follow the vata-pacifying diet from fall through winter and early spring, the pitta-pacifying diet from late spring through summer.

For vata-kapha:
Follow the vata-pacifying diet from summer through fall, the kapha-pacifying diet from winter through spring.

For pitta-kapha:
Follow the pitta-pacifying diet from late spring through fall, the kapha-pacifying diet from winter through early spring.

For tri-doshic (vata-pitta-kapha):
Change diet according to the season: vata-pacifying diet during the fall, kapha-pacifying diet during winter to early spring, pitta-pacifying diet from late spring through summer.

Vata

Vata food should be:
- very nourishing
- cooked
- warm
- moist
- mildly spiced

  Meals should be consumed at regular hours to alleviate the vata tendency toward hypoglycemia and nervousness. This type of food and routine will counteract vata's dry, cold, light, agitated, dispersing, mobile nature.

Grains: Well-cooked oats and rice are very healthy for vatas. Buckwheat, corn, millet, and rye are also recommended, but only when cooked with extra water; otherwise, these grains can be drying to vatas or in vata conditions.

Vegetables: Vatas do better with cooked than raw vegetables. Hard vegetables like celery are better for vatas when juiced. Tomato sauce (not whole tomatoes) with spices added is okay from time to time. Asparagus, beets, carrots, celery, garlic, okra, onions, parsnip, radish, rutabaga, turnip, sweet potato, and water chestnut are all fine. Broccoli and other vegetables of the *brassica* family may be added to stews and soups, or steamed well with a spice-and-oil dressing to counteract gas formation. Raw salads and vegetables may be too cooling and therefore hard for vatas to digest, so vata people are advised to stay away from them unless the digestive processes are quite healthy.

Fruits: Most fruits, excepting the astringent ones or any unripe fruit, are fine. If raw fruit causes digestive problems, take the fruit stewed with cinnamon or other mild spices. Vatas should have no dried fruit unless reconstituted; plain dried fruit dries the vata person out too much. Apricot, banana, cherry, dates, figs, grapes, grapefruit, lemon, limes, mango, papaya, peaches, pears, persimmons, pineapple, plums, oranges, and tangerines are all fine.

Meats: Meats tend to ground and nourish vatas or vata conditions, but remember that heavy meats can dull the mind. Purchase organic meat whenever possible, and choose chicken and fish over beef and pork.

Legumes: Mung beans are best for vata. Vatas may have soy products in moderation if there is no consequent discomfort.

Nuts and Seeds: Vatas may eat nuts in moderation—not big handfuls of them! Peanuts are not recommended, because they clot the blood. Nut butters are better, again in moderation. Almonds (without skins), black walnuts, cashews, Brazil nuts, coconut, pecans, pine nuts, pistachios, macadamia nuts, flax seed, halvah, psyllium, pumpkin, sesame- and sunflower seed are all fine.

Oils: Sesame is the best oil for vata, while safflower oil is the worst. Olive oil, ghee (see glossary), and almond oil are also recommended.

Dairy: All dairy is good for vatas who are not allergic to it. Hard cheeses, however, should be cooked into a more liquid form. Lassi, a beverage made of yogurt blended with water and spices (see glossary), especially helps vatas.

Sweet: Vatas may use sweeteners in moderation. A healthy sweetener on the market is Sucanat®, made from the dehydrated juice of organic sugarcane.

Spices: Spices will help with digestion and counteract gas, but they are drying—so use them only in vata-pacifying foods, or as tea. Especially recommended are anise, fennel, cloves, pepper, bay, orange peel, oregano, rosemary, garlic, ginger, cumin, cinnamon, hingashtak (a combination of herbs for gas and digestion that may be purchased at East Indian markets), cardamom, and nutmeg.

Herbs: Building herbs for vata constitutions or conditions include:

    codonopsis (*Codonopsis pilosula*; Chinese *Dang shen*)
    American ginseng (*Panax quinquefolium*)
    dong quai (*Angelica sinensis*)

angelica (*archangelica*)
marshmallow root (*althea officinalis*)
aloe vera juice or gel (*aloe barbadensis*)—mix with a pinch
    of ginger to counteract aloe's cold nature
shatavari (*Asparagus racemosus*)
ashwagandha or winter cherry (*withania somnifera*)
slippery elm (*Ulmus fulva*)
licorice root (*Glycyrrhiza glabra*)

Herbs for Elimination:

triphala (*Myrobalan*)
psyllium husks (*Plantago psyllium*)

Herbs for the Nerves:

basil (*Ocinum spp.*)
biota seeds (*Biota orientalis*)
valerian (*Valeriana officinalis*)
jujube dates (*ziziphus jujuba*)
oatstraw (*Avena Sativa*)

The preceding herbs may be mixed with the cooling, bitter
nervine herbs such as skullcap and passion flower. Combining
warmer-energy herbs with cooling herbs will counteract the
cooling quality.

Other Vata-Pacifying Herbs:

orange peel (*Citrus aurantium*)
fresh ginger (*zingiber officinalis*)
fennel (*foeniculum vulgare*)
hawthorn (*crataegus oxycantha*)
sassafras (*sassafras albidum*)
sarsaparilla (*smilax spp.*)
lemon grass (*cymbopogon citratus*)
rose hips (*rosa spp.*)

Vatas are prone to addiction, so all add[...]
drugs, alcohol, cigarettes, caffeine, white su[...]
should be avoided.

Vata is calmed down by regular application o[...]
the following blend:

2 oz. sesame oil
2 oz. almond oil
10 drops lavender essential oil
10 drops rose geranium essential oil

Mix ingredients together and use daily all over the body.
The feet may be massaged at night with this formula to allow
for more restful sleep.

Pitta

Pitta food should be:
- cool in nature
- very mildly spiced
- sweet in taste
- small amounts of bitter and astringent

The food should not be too spicy, hot, sour, or salty.
Pittas should avoid meat and alcohol. Steamed or stir-fried vegetables are recommended, and if the pitta person has good digestion, raw vegetables may be eaten as well. Mild spices are
fine, and the atmosphere for a meal should be calm. (Pittas
should not eat while conducting business meetings, nor should
they engage in heavy discussions over dinner.) In general, people
with the pitta constitution will do best on a vegetarian diet.

Grains: barley, rice, oats, wheat, amaranth, dry cereal,
couscous, tapioca.

Vegetables: All vegetables that are sweet and bitter are fine;
sour vegetables such as tomatoes, as well as pungent vegetables

...ctive substances—
...ar, et cetera—
...oils. I use

...lic, should be avoided. Steamed white ...ay occasionally; red or purple onions ...ers. Pittas can have asparagus, arti- ...ccoli, Brussels sprouts, cabbage, cau- ...er, celery, green beans, leafy greens, ...a, black olives, peas, parsley, pota- ...atoes, pumpkin, wheat grass, and

Fruits: sweet fruits are okay; avoid sour. Papaya has too great a heating quality, and bananas have a souring effect in the body. Figs and sweet grapes are especially good for pittas, as are sweet apples, avocado, berries, cherries, coconut, dates, figs, limes, melons, pears, plums, pomegranates, prunes, and raisins. Sweet oranges and pineapples are tolerated by some pittas, but others may find them irritating.

Flesh Foods: Pittas should avoid eating seafood because it is "heating" in nature and tends to cause allergies. Fresh-water fish would be a better choice. Flesh foods generally encourage pitta aggression and irritability. Meats that tend to be less aggravating for pitta are white meat of chicken and turkey, rabbit, and venison.

Legumes: Pittas can have all beans, including aduki, black and white beans, chickpeas, kidney beans, lentils, lima and mung beans, mung dahl, navy beans, peas, pinto beans, soy products, split peas, and tempeh.

Nuts and Seeds: Pittas should avoid nuts for the most part because they are too oily. Peanuts are not recommended because they clot the blood. Small quantities (1 tbsp. or less) of walnuts, pecans, Brazil nuts, cashews (occassionally) are okay. Large amounts would have an unbalancing effect on pitta. Nuts that are most beneficial to pitta are almonds (soaked and peeled), coconut, pumpkin seeds (unsalted), sunflower seeds, flax, and pine nuts.

Oils: Pitta can use the following oils internally: sunflower, ghee (see glossary), canola, olive. Externally, pitta will find the use of coconut oil quite cooling.

Dairy: Pitta can have unsalted butter, soft unsalted cheese, cottage cheese, milk, the yogurt beverage lassi, and ghee (see glossary).

Sweet: The sweet taste cools off pitta. It is best to avoid large amounts of molasses and long-term use of honey, as both have a heating effect. Pittas can use fruit-juice sweetener, barley malt, maple syrup, rice syrup, Sucanat®, or turbinado sugar.

Spices: fresh basil, cardamom, cilantro, cinnamon, coriander, dill, fennel, fresh ginger, mints, orange peel, saffron, turmeric, and small amounts of cumin, black pepper, and vanilla are all recommended.

Herbs: The herbs listed below are best for pitta and pitta conditions such as heat and inflammation. Herbs with a cooling, sweet, bitter, and astringent energy are best for pitta.

Herb Beverages for Pitta and Pitta Conditions:
> catnip (*nepeta cataria*)
> alfalfa (*medicago sativa*)
> violets (*viola spp.*)
> mints (*mentha spp.*)
> chickweed (*stellaria media*)
> nettles (*urtica urens*)
> raspberry (*Rubus spp.*)
> cleavers (*galium spp.*)
> grain "coffee" substitutes (Pero, Cafix, Inca)
> cinnamon, in moderation (*cinnamomum zeylanicum*)

cardamom, in moderation (*elettaria cardamomum*)
strawberry leaf (*fragaria spp.*)

Herbs for Calming and Relaxing:
lavender (*lavandula spp.*)
rose petals (*rosa spp.*)
skullcap (*scutellaria spp.*)
passion flower (*passiflora incarnata*)
biota seeds (*biota orientalis*)
zizyphus seeds (*zizyphus spinosa*)
chamomile (*matricaria chamomila*)
lemon balm (*melissa officinalis*)
oatstraw (*avena sativa*)

Herbs for the Liver (Pitta Organ):
barberry bark (*berberis spp.*)
dandelion leaf and root (*taraxacum vulgare*)
fennel (*foeniculum vulgare*)
gentian (*gentiana spp.*)
hops (*humulus lupulus*)
milk thistle seed (*silybum marianum*)
sarsaparilla (*smilax spp.*)
burdock root and seeds (*arctium lappa*)
red clover (*trifolium pratense*)
yellow dock (*rumex crispus*)
turmeric (*curcuma longa*)

Herbs to Strengthen and Build Energy in a Pitta Person:
aloe vera (*aloe spp.*)
licorice (*glycyrrhiza glabra*)
marshmallow root (*althea officinalis*)
peony root (*paeonia lactiflora*)
comfrey (*symphytum officinale*)
slippery elm (*ulmus fulva*)
shitavari (*asparagus racemosus*)

Herbs for Elimination:
    For loose stool:
        amalaki (*emblica officinalis*)
        psyllium husks (*plantago psyllium*)

These two herbs work well in combination with one another. Mix equal parts and take two "00" capsules at bedtime.
    For constipation:
        prunes
        cascara sagrada

Herbs for Infection and Inflammation (Pitta Conditions):
    echinacea (*echinacea purpurea–angustifolia pallida*)
    goldenseal (*hydrastis canadensis*)
    Oregon grape root (*mahonia repens*)
    usnea or lichen (*Usnea longissima* and others)
    boneset (*eupatorium perfoliatum*)

Kapha

Kapha food should be:
- warm, dry, light in nature
- emphasize pungent, bitter, astringent tastes
- spicy
- vegetable-rich

Kaphas and those with kapha conditions need to avoid or minimize the sweet, sour, and salty tastes. Fried or greasy foods are extremely detrimental.

Grains: Hot, drying grains like buckwheat and millet are good for kapha, as are barley, rice, corn, dry cereals, couscous, crackers (unsalted), muesli, dry oats, and polenta. Breads should be avoided unless toasted.

Vegetables: Kaphas can eat most vegetables. Not recommended are sweet potatoes, pumpkin, zucchini, winter and spaghetti squash, raw tomatoes, and cucumbers.

Fruits: Avoid sweet and sour fruits. Dried fruits are okay. Cold fruit juice may be mucus-forming, so take juice warm in small amounts.

Flesh: Meats are best roasted or broiled in small amounts: white chicken, eggs, fresh-water fish, shrimp, turkey (white meat), rabbit.

Legumes: Aduki, black beans, chickpeas, lentils, lima, navy, peas, pinto, soy products, tempeh, white beans.

Nuts and Seeds: Avoid nuts. Popcorn with no salt or butter is fine, as are sunflower seeds and pumpkin seeds.

Oils: In general, avoid oils, but when necessary use corn, canola, sunflower, ghee (see glossary), and almond.

Dairy: Avoid for the most part, although very small amounts of unsalted butter or ghee (see glossary), cottage cheese from skimmed milk, goat's cheese (unsalted), goat's milk, the yogurt beverage lassi (see glossary), and soy milk (without added oil) are okay.

Sweeteners: Raw honey, sparingly.

Spices: All spices are good, except salt. One spice in particular is very good for kapha: trikatu (see glossary), which breaks up mucus and facilitates digestion.

Herbs: building herbs for kapha include:
aloe vera juice/gel (*aloe spp.*)

angelica archangelica
elecampane (*Inula spp.*)
Siberian ginseng (*eleutherococcus senticosus*)
dong quai (*angelica sinensis*)
ashwagandha (*withania somnifera*)

Often, kaphas do not need building as much as stimulating herbs, such as spices, to break up congestion in the body. The tonic herbs listed above—many of which have a warming energy and help move energy—are recommended for kaphas who feel weak and run-down.

Herbs for Cleansing:

barberry (*berberis spp.*)
bayberry bark (*myrica cerifera*)
cascara sagrada
hops (*humulus lupulus*)
dandelion (*taraxacum vulgare*)
burdock (*arctium lappa*)
Oregon grape root (*mahonia repens*)
milk thistle seed (*silybum marianum*)
turmeric (*curcuma longa*)
juniper berries (*juniperus spp.*)
eucalyptus (*eucalyptus globulus*)
fennel (*foeniculum vulgare*)

Herbs for Mucous Conditions:

elecampane (*inula spp.*)
ginger (*zingiber officinalis*)
horehound (*marrubium vulgare*)
hyssop (*hyssopus officinalis*)
thyme (*thymus vulgaris*)
garlic (*allium sativum*)
grindelia (*grindelia robusta*)

marshmallow root (*althea officinalis*)—helps to liquify mucus; small amounts may be added to cough formulas; excess amounts may increase kapha and ama (toxins)

licorice (*glycyrrhiza glabra*)—small amounts of licorice root may be added to help liquify mucus; excess amounts of licorice may create water retention in some people

Other Herbs for Kapha:
alfalfa (*medicago sativa*)
chamomile (*anthemis nobilis*)
lavender (*lavandula spp.*)
lemon grass (*cymbopogon citratus*)
chicory (*cichorium intybus*)
hibiscus (*hibiscus rosa sinensis*)
lemon balm (*melissa officinalis*)
mints (*mentha*)
red clover (*trifolium pratense*)
grain beverages

Food Quality

For many thousands of years of Ayurvedic practice, there was no concern about whether food was organically grown or free of chemicals. In modern times, we should take pains to find out whether our food has been contaminated by antibiotics, growth hormones, drugs, pesticides, or herbicides. Such drugs are easily transferred to human beings through diet, creating a disruption of the beneficial flora in the digestive tract and eventually compromising the immune system.

The FDA permits milk to contain a certain concentration of 80 different antibiotics, used on dairy cows to prevent udder infections. Plant foods grown with petrochemical fertilizers are very low in mineral content; they may look pretty, but they do not contain the same level of vitality as organic produce. Such pesticide and herbicide residues also create adverse reactions in the body-mind.

White sugar is deranging to everyone—vatas, pittas, kaphas—so don't use it. Two other dangerous additives, becoming more and more prevalent in our foods, are Nutrasweet and MSG. Both of these substances can aggravate the liver and nervous system, and should be avoided whenever possible.

It is important for each of us to try our best to purchase clean produce, dairy products, and meat. For readers who do not have resources for such products close by, there are many natural-foods cooperatives around the country that will ship foods free of drugs and pesticides to different locales. I also feel that, if possible, we should all try growing some of our own food and herbs, which will enhance our sense of responsibility for what we eat, and get us in tune with the seasons and nature.

Due to the excessive consumption of antibiotics (whether prescribed by a doctor, or in milk and meats), cortisone, birth-control pills, and sugar, many people have had the favorable flora in their digestive tracts destroyed. Digestion therefore may be irregular, with excessive gas, bloating, malabsorption of nutrients, and an overgrowth of yeast. In my practice I have found it necessary to advise people to replace the good flora with acidophilus supplementation. Some people have had to stay on high doses of acidophilus—one teaspoon of the powder three times per day for six months to one year—in order to handle their yeast and digestive disruptions. As a preventative treatment, acidophilus may be taken for one month twice in a year.

Life Cycles

Times of the Day

Morning, after sunrise, is the kapha time of the day. People with a mucous condition will have more mucus flowing at this time. There may be a tendency to sluggishness, as the digestive fires may not have been awakened yet. A mild, spicy herbal tea—such as fresh ginger tea, or cinnamon blended with cardamom and orange peel—is appropriate for the morning. Stay away from cold juice and cheese, which will only create more mucus.

Evening after sunset is the other kapha time of the day. Again, one should be careful not to eat kapha-type foods, such as cheese and ice cream; otherwise, mucus may accumulate and create difficulty the following morning.

Pitta time is the afternoon, when the sun is high in the sky. The digestive fires are also high, and this is the best time for the main meal of the day. For those with pitta conditions, it is best to stay away from alcohol, spices, and other heating foods during the noon hour; otherwise, there may be some provoking of burning sensations.

Eleven p.m. until around one or two a.m. is the other pitta time of day. People with gallstones or liver problems may experience discomfort at this time because of the increased acid flow. It is therefore best to avoid acidic, spicy foods before bed; otherwise, there may be acid indigestion and other burning sensations later in the night. Try having a cup of mild, calming tea before bed for a restful sleep. A good blend is passion flower, chamomile, and spearmint.

Sunrise and sunset, and the hours just before, are the vata times of the day. Many people with vata disturbances and worries will wake up around three a.m. and start to think about their own problems or the problems of the world. This may also be a time when disturbing dreams occur. Many yogis will get up at three or four a.m. and practice meditation because this is a good time for tapping into deeper inspiration.

Sunset and sunrise are both times of great transition. Remember, vata governs our aspiration to higher consciousness. Many cultures around the world pray and meditate at these times in order to focus on the divine principles that govern life.

Seasons of the Year

Each season, with its characteristic weather conditions, expresses a certain constitution. If we become aware of the different qualities, we can moderate our activities to harmonize with the season.

Fall	Winter–Early Spring	Late Spring–Summer
(vata season)	(kapha season)	(pitta season)
windy	cold	hot
dry	damp	humid
cold	foggy	bright

Vata people and conditions will be most affected by dry, windy, cold environments; they must closely follow the vata-pacifying diet and stay out of the cold. Pitta people and conditions will be affected during hot weather; during the hot months they must stay out of the direct sun and eat cooling foods. Kapha people and conditions will be affected adversely during cold, damp times; they need to eat spicy, dry foods during those times, so as to reduce accumulation of mucus and congestion.

Seasons of Our Lives

Just as the seasons change throughout the year, human beings experience different seasons in their lives:

Kapha	**Pitta**	**Vata**
(childhood)	(adulthood)	(seniors)
development	production	detachment
building	create/transform	completions
(anabolism)	(metabolism)	(catabolism)
mucous conditions	heat conditions	bone conditions

Underlying our constitution and our imbalances are the seasons of our lives. During the kapha-building stage of life, children may experience mucous conditions and therefore need to have limits imposed on the amount of dairy they take in, or at least have their milk gently boiled with a pinch of cardamom, cinnamon, and ginger. (These spices counteract milk's mucus-producing qualities.) They will also need foods that help them to build physically and mentally.

During the adult years, people often experience inflammatory heart and blood diseases. At this phase, we require herbs and foods that help keep the digestion strong and energy moving: hawthorn berries for the heart, dandelion for the liver, marshmallow root for the kidneys.

In the senior years, bodies no longer regenerate as easily and there may be a breakdown of various systems. Seniors often experience vata conditions such as coldness, arthritis, and poor elimination. They need foods and a lifestyle that are nourishing and calming. Daily applications of oil to their bodies will help with dryness. Herbs such as ginkgo will stimulate blood circulation in the brain, which will offset any tendencies toward memory loss. Other helpful herbs are ashwagandha for building and marshmallow root for lubricating the inner organs.

Knowing that we are in a certain season of our lives, we can acknowledge and accept the changes that we are experiencing and, with greater awareness, take the appropriate steps to enhance our physical and spiritual evolution.

Simple Remedies for Common Ailments

Digestive Disturbances

Vata-type digestive disturbance:
- gas
- bloating
- variable appetite
- constipation
- insomnia
- palpitations
- nervousness

Follow the vata-pacifying diet and routine. Try to live your life rhythmically, eliminating any erratic or chaotic ways. This applies especially to mealtimes. Do not skip meals, then eat frantically because of extreme hunger. Do not eat while agitated, while working, or while running from place to place. Create an atmosphere of quiet and calm at mealtimes. Avoid sugary foods like cookies and ice cream, or dry foods like crackers or rice cakes. Have some spiced tea—e.g., ginger, fennel, cumin, cardamom or cinnamon—during the day and after meals. Cook foods with an emphasis on culinary spices. The herbal combination called *hingashtak*, which may be purchased from most Indian markets (see distributors listed in back of this guide), is recommended. One-eighth to one-quarter teaspoon may be added to vegetables as they sauté to enhance digestion and absorption. A cup of ginger tea may be helpful after meals as well—or try chewing fennel seeds.

Pitta-type digestive disturbance:
- heartburn
- hyperacidity
- diarrhea or loose stool
- irritability
- gas
- burning sensation when excreting
- rash or redness of the skin

The pitta-pacifying diet should be followed, with strict avoidance of acidic and spicy foods. Try cooling carminatives (herbs that relieve intestinal gas, pain, and stomach distention), such as mints, fennel and coriander. Bitter herbs are also appropriate. Try this bitter combination:

2 parts gentian	1 part fennel
2 parts dandelion	1/8 part dry ginger
1 part Oregon grape	1/8 part licorice

This may be taken as an alcoholic extract (tincture), in capsules, or in a tea. It is best to take bitters 15 minutes before meals, or as burning sensations occur.

A tea of cumin, coriander, and fennel is also helpful. Mix equal parts of the three herbs together, put one teaspoon of the combination in a cup of boiling water and let it steep for 10 minutes. Drink after meals.

A simple tea of dandelion, mint, and licorice may be helpful as well. Aloe vera juice is also very cooling and alleviates burning.

Demulcent herbs (herbs that soothe and protect the internal membranes) may be brewed into a tea, along with some of the bitters. The following is a good combination:

marshmallow root	mint
dandelion leaf	licorice root

Mix one ounce each of these herbs together. Take one tablespoon of the combination and place it in boiling water. Let steep for 20 minutes, strain, and drink as needed.

Kapha-type digestive disturbance:

If we eat lots of foods that are mucus-forming—such as ice cream and cheese, fatty fried foods, or rancid foods—we may experience kapha digestive problems. Symptoms include:

- nausea and vomiting
- mucus in throat or chest after meals
- lethargy after meals
- general congestion

The kapha-pacifying regimen must be followed, and no cold food or drink should be taken. Do not overeat, and keep the diet simple: soups, steamed vegetables, grains. Morning and evening are the kapha times of the day. There will be a greater tendency for the body to create mucus at these times. Therefore, do not eat cold, mucus-forming foods—milk, cheese, ice cream, yogurt, et cetera—in the mornings or evenings. Hot spices are appropriate treatment for kapha disturbances. The following are kapha-pacifying spices:

- cayenne
- dry ginger
- pepper
- cinnamon
- cloves
- cardamom
- Yogi tea (available at most health stores)

Bitters may also be taken before meals when kapha is disturbed. Remember, the bitter, pungent, and astringent tastes are pacifying to kapha conditions. You may use the recipe for bitters listed under pitta digestive disturbances; however, a little extra ginger and even a pinch of cayenne will make the formula even better for the kapha condition.

Colds and Flu

Vata-type cold and flu

Symptoms include:
- dry cough
- dry nose or throat
- clear mucus, but scanty
- insomnia
- loss of voice due to dryness
- chills
- erratic fever
- fear or anxiety

The treatment for the vata-type cold and flu is basically to heat up and moisten the sufferer. This is best accomplished by using warming spices such as cinnamon, cardamom, ginger, garlic, and Yogi tea. Helpful demulcent herbs include licorice, marshmallow, comfrey, and slippery elm. A warm bath with the addition of one-quarter cup powdered ginger will help alleviate chills; a heating pad or hot-water bottle on the kidneys may also give some relief. The sufferer should stay warm and out of drafts. Generally, the vata-pacifying regimen should be adhered to, with an emphasis on simple, warming foods. Hard-to-digest food such as nuts and dairy should be avoided. If the nasal passages are dry and sore, then three or four drops sesame oil in the nostrils will help to lubricate the area.

To boost the immune system, take the herb echinacea mixed with a little licorice root, one dropperful of the tincture or two capsules every two hours during acute stages. Licorice root will help counteract the dizzy feelings some people—especially vata types—experience when taking echinacea. Cut the dose back as symptoms subside.

Pitta-type cold and flu

Symptoms include:
- high fever
- burning sensation
- heat
- yellow or green discharges
- sore throat
- agitation

Follow the pitta-pacifying diet, but avoid meat and dairy. If the sufferer has an appetite, offer mild soups and broths. Cooling herbs such as burdock, elder flowers, peppermint, yarrow, lemon balm, and mints will also be helpful. Echinacea and goldenseal may be taken every two hours until symptoms subside. These herbs are very bitter and will enhance the body's healing capacities. Bitters reduce heat in the body and are very cleansing to the system. (For a list of bitters, see the pitta food list under "Dietary Recommendations.")

To ease a sore throat, add about four or five drops tea-tree oil to one-half cup warm water and gargle. This can be done a number of times throughout the day, and it is okay to swallow after gargling. Tea tree is an excellent antiseptic and antibiotic. Echinacea and/or goldenseal extract may be used in this manner as well.

To help break a fever, make a strong tea of the following herbs:

elder flowers
peppermint
yarrow

Mix equal parts of the herbs together. Take one heaping tablespoon of the combination and let it steep in a cup of boiling water for 15 minutes. Drink up to three cups per day. To induce sweating, you may want to wrap yourself in a blanket while drinking this tea.

Kapha-type cold and flu

Symptoms include:

- low-grade fever
- loss of appetite
- excess mucus, clear or white in color
- excess salivation
- mucus in stool or urine
- lethargy or heavy feeling
- possible chilled feeling

If there is an appetite, then follow the kapha-pacifying diet. The food should be very simple, mainly soups and broths. Do not take heavy foods such as cheese, meat, or bread.

About one-quarter to one-half teaspoon trikatu paste in hot water may be taken as a tea, as needed, throughout the day. The bitter herbs listed in the section on pitta digestive disturbances may be taken as well. Strong ginger tea usually helps quite a bit: grate about three tablespoons of fresh ginger and let it gently steep in two cups of water for 15 minutes or so. Add honey and lemon to taste.

Echinacea and/or goldenseal may be taken every two hours. Echinacea helps activate the immune system; goldenseal cleanses the mucous membranes and counteracts inflammation. Continue until the symptoms subside, then cut the dose back to three times per day.

If the sufferer feels chilled, a ginger bath may be appropriate. Add one-quarter cup of ginger powder to the tub. Soak for 15 minutes or longer.

Coughs

A cough with phlegm and congestion usually indicates a kapha disorder. The kapha-pacifying diet must be accompanied by strict avoidance of iced drinks, fruit juices, soda, fried foods, cheese, milk, dairy, and white sugar. Such cold and "heavy" foods will increase mucus throughout the body. On the other hand, warm, spicy teas may be taken freely throughout the day. Ginger tea with honey will be especially therapeutic. Many times a short fast is helpful when one has a cough, cold, or flu.

A simple home remedy for relieving congestion is to chop three onions and steam them until they are soft. Place the onions between two layers of cheesecloth, then place the warm mass on the chest or upper back. Cover the area with a dry cloth and keep it warm with a hot-water bottle or heating pad for 30 minutes or longer. Onions have natural antibiotic properties and are a tremendous aid against pneumonia, lung infection, asthma, and mucous congestion due to colds.

Eucalyptus essential oil may be mixed with olive or sesame oils, 10 drops of the essential oil per ounce of base oil. Shake well, then rub directly on the chest or back to relieve lung congestion. The aroma will also help clear sinuses.

Warming expectorant herbs

The following herbs have a spicy, "warm" nature and help in the treatment of coughing, vomiting, asthma, and other mucous conditions. They help to remove energy-channel blockages in the body that may cause nerve damage, strokes, paralysis, and tremors:

- yerba santa
- platycodon
- osha root
- hyssop
- lovage
- thyme
- elecampane
- basil

Antispasmodic herbs

The following herbs, which are used mainly for conditions of cold with dampness (kapha) or heat with dampness (pitta), will help with cough spasms that leave a person exhausted or in pain, and may be combined with some of the other herbs in this section:

- wild lettuce
- mullein
- wild cherry bark
- apricot seed
- coltsfoot
- anise seeds
- lobelia

Demulcent herbs for coughs

The herbs in this category are used to help soften mucus for elimination. They also help to cool and lubricate inflamed mucous membranes:

- marshmallow root
- licorice root
- comfrey root

The following formula tastes nasty, but will also help to break up mucus:

2 parts elecampane
1 part thyme leaves
1 part grindelia
1 part Mormon tea (American ephedra)
1/2 part licorice root
1/4 part anise seeds

Gently simmer one ounce of this combination for 20 minutes in three cups of water, strain, and drink 1/2 cup of the tea four or five times per day. Add honey if desired.

Vata-Type Coughs

Coughs may be the result of imbalances in the other humors, as well. The vata-type cough will be dry with very little expectoration. When a coughing spasm occurs, there may be pain in the chest, heart, and throat. The treatment adds to the vata-pacifying diet demulcent herbs such as licorice root, marshmallow root, comfrey root, and ophiopogon, which are nourishing and moistening to dry lungs. They will also lubricate, soften, and release any mucus that may have hardened and become stuck.

Mild spices such as cardamom and ginger may be added to the demulcent herbs. Spices bring warmth to the lungs and move energy. Again, strictly follow the vata-pacifying diet and lifestyle, but stay away from hard-to-digest foods such as dairy and nuts.

Try the following vata cough formula:

2 parts comfrey leaves
1 part elecampane
1 part licorice root
1/4 part anise seeds
1/4 part ginger
pinch of cloves

Let one tablespoon of the herbal combination steep in a cup of boiling water for 20–30 minutes. Strain and drink 1/4 cup four times per day. To enhance the tea's soothing properties, add honey.

Pitta-Type Coughs

With the pitta-type cough, there will be yellow, green, or blood-streaked phlegm. There may be burning sensations in the lungs, accompanied by fever, thirst, and dryness. Antibiotic herbs—goldenseal, echinacea and/or usnea—should be taken every hour or two. Demulcent herbs, such as licorice root and marshmallow root, will help cool off and soften mucus in the bronchial tubes and lungs. Other cooling expectorant herbs include:

- comfrey leaves
- horehound
- mullein
- coltsfoot

The following formula is very good for the pitta-type cough:

1 part coltsfoot
1 part comfrey
1 part mullein
1 part yarrow
1/4 part lobelia
1/4 part ginger
1/2 part licorice root

This formula does not taste very good, but it is effective. One ounce of the herb combination is gently simmered in three cups of water, keeping the lid on the pot. Strain and drink 1/2 cup four or five times a day.

The onion plaster described at the beginning of this section may also prove useful. Follow the pitta-pacifying diet, but also eliminate dairy, bread, and sweets. Do not take any cold, iced, or mucus-forming foods.

Sore Throat

Sore throats are oftentimes a complication of a flu or cold, and are of several different types.

The vata-type sore throat feels dry and scratchy. The voice may have a hoarse quality. There won't be extreme pain upon swallowing, nor will there be much of a feeling of "thickness." A simple but effective remedy is to make a paste out of slippery-elm powder mixed with raw honey. Take one-quarter teaspoon of this combination and let it melt in your mouth.

Slippery elm has a demulcent quality that will help soothe the throat. The honey also will help to coat a dry throat.

A tea may be made of the following herbs:

- 2 parts slippery elm
- 2 parts licorice root
- 1 part comfrey leaf
- 1 part fennel seeds
- 1/8 part orange peel

Take a teaspoon of this combination, place it in a muslin tea bag and let it steep in a cup of boiling water for five minutes. (Slippery elm is sold as a powder, but if this is put directly into the water, it will make the tea rather slimy.) You may prefer to make a paste out of this formula rather than take it as a tea. Powder all the herbs, then add honey until the consistency is that of a thick paste. Store the paste in a glass jar and carry it with you wherever you go for instant herbal therapy.

The Ayurvedic herb shatavari will also ease a dry throat. Add one teaspoon of the herb to raw milk or soy milk, and gently boil for fifteen minutes. Add honey to taste. Ghee (see glossary) or sesame oil also may be taken internally to soothe an irritated throat.

Painful strep-like conditions of the throat usually indicate a pitta-type condition. Antibiotic herbs—such as goldenseal, echinacea and usnea (a lichen)—are appropriate for this condition. Take one dropperful every two hours. The dose is kept high until the symptoms have subsided, at which point the dose may be slowly decreased.

I have also found that gargling with lemon juice and honey mixed in water is helpful. The antiseptic quality of the lemon will help kill bacteria, and honey soothes the throat. I have also recommended a tea-tree gargle for sore throats. Add four or five drops of tea tree oil to warm water, shake well, and gargle. If sore throat is accompanied by dryness, try the demulcent formulas listed above for the vata condition. If the sufferer has an appetite, serve only broths and soups of a pitta-pacifying nature (see "Dietary Recommendations").

If the sore throat is also accompanied by mucus, which indicates a complication of pitta and/or kapha, then the following warming herbs may be used in various formulas:

- sage
- bayberry
- turmeric
- garlic
- cloves

Garlic stimulates the metabolism, is very warming, and is good for breaking up mucus. It is also an effective antibiotic for staphylococcus, streptococcus, salmonella, and other bacteria resistant to standard antibiotic drugs. Sage may be used as a gargle to break up mucus that is lodged in the throat and larynx. The expectorant herbs listed in the "Cough" section of this chapter may be employed as well.

Nervous Debility, Insomnia and Anxiety

Nervous exhaustion and its accompanying symptoms are a sure sign of stress. There are many herbal remedies for nervous exhaustion, but the biggest consideration is lifestyle choices. Causes of nervous exhaustion, insomnia, and anxiety include:

- poor food combinations
- too much sugar
- drinking coffee and other stimulating substances
- skipping meals
- undernourishing meals
- lack of routine in life
- excess exercise, which can deplete the body of energy
- no exercise at all
- heavy use of computers and other electronic devices

- excess exposure to mass media
- overwork
- loud music and noises
- excessive sexual activity

As my teacher once said, "We are all suffering from global nervousness and anxiety." If you are suffering from nervous exhaustion, try your best to deal with some of the causes listed above. This will help to create a stronger basis for herbal healing.

Insomnia and anxiety are commonly an aggravated vata condition. Symptoms include:
- fear
- worry
- heart palpitations
- difficulty breathing
- inability to concentrate
- poor digestion
- lack of appetite
- ungroundedness
- emotional emptiness
- eating binges
- difficulty falling asleep
- disturbing dreams, especially of flying or falling

Rhythm and routine help to calm vata down. Try to eat at regular hours. The food should be nourishing and vata-pacifying. Stimulating herbs and substances, such as coffee, black tea, sugar, and Chinese ephedra (ma huang), should be avoided. Each evening before bed the feet should be massaged with almond or sesame oil. A few drops of lavender or rose essential oil may be added to the massage oil to enhance its calming properties. A time of meditation and self-reflection should be reserved for each morning and evening. Chanting a calming mantra or the repeating of a positive affirmation will help. Most people have unconscious mantras they repeat all day long, such as "I don't have enough money," "I'm miserable", et cetera. Repeating more positive statements can change our inner as well as our outer reality.

Vata-Type Nervous Debility

For vata-type nervous exhaustion and/or insomnia, the following Western herb formula will be helpful:

2 parts valerian
1 part skullcap
1 part oatstraw
1 part hops
1 part rose petals
1 part gotu kola
1 part marshmallow
1 part licorice root
(If you can find biota seed in bulk, add it to the formula.)

Take one tablespoon of the combination and add it to a cup of boiling water. Let it steep for 10 minutes and drink three cups per day. You may also purchase the herbs in powder form and fill up "00" sized capsules. Take two capsules three to six times per day as needed. This formula is not only calming but nourishing, which is essential for grounding high vata.

Valerian helps to clear vata from the nerve channels, and eases spasms and cramping. Because valerian contains a large amount of the earth element, it helps calm hysteria and ease vertigo. Its pungent taste also aids in digestion and alleviates gas. (The Ayurvedic herb jatamamsi is in the same family as valerian and may be used in its place. It does not create as dulling a sensation as valerian sometimes will.)

It is important to strengthen the digestive capacities of an individual when he or she is manifesting disease tendencies. If our food is not being digested and absorbed properly, then we will continue to feel run down. For example, the vata person may experience a wasting away of nerve tissue due to poor digestion and absorption, which eventually results in malnutrition. Add some mild spices to the diet to help increase *agni* (digestive fires). Make sure the food is chewed well and that the mealtime is peaceful.

Pitta-Type Nervous Debility

Pitta-type insomnia and nervous exhaustion is usually due to turbulent emotions such as anger, hatred, resentment, and the desire for revenge. Many times, pittas will be unable to sleep following an argument, after meeting a deadline, or during extreme heat conditions such as fevers or sunbathing. Sleep may be agitated and filled with violent dreams, which leaves pittas tired in the morning. Some of the symptoms may be the same as for vata, but they will carry more heat, more burning sensations, more agitation, and more emotional outbursts. The causes for these situations may include:
- excessive willfulness
- excessive competition
- eating hot, stimulating foods
- too much exposure to sun and heat
- high fevers
- wanting too much control over situations
- watching violent movies or TV shows

The remedy for this condition is to follow the pitta-pacifying diet, i.e., avoid excess spices, including salty and sour tastes. Meditations by a source of water or in the moonlight will help cool off heated emotions. Cooling colors and calming scents may also be helpful for pitta. Massage the feet at night with coconut oil and add a few drops of sandalwood essential oil to enhance its cooling properties. A drop of sandalwood oil on the "third eye" will cool off the mind as well.

A good Western herb formula for pitta is equal parts:
- skullcap
- gotu kola
- passion flower
- hops
- spearmint
- lemon balm
- St. John's wort
- rose petals
- licorice root

Take one tablespoon of the mixture and let it steep in one cup of boiling water until the water cools to room temperature. Strain and drink three cups per day or as needed. Or powder the herbs and fill "00" size capsules with the mixture. Take two capsules three to six times per day as needed.

For depression and hopelessness, the following formula is helpful:
- 2 parts oatstraw
- 1 part St. John's wort
- 2 parts lemon balm
- 1 part rose petals
- 1/4 part licorice

This can be made into a tea, one tablespoon of the herb combination to a cup of boiling water. Let steep for 20 minutes, strain, and drink three cups per day. This formula may be used for pitta and kapha constitutions. The vata person may want to add some jatamamsi and a little extra licorice root.

Kapha-Type Nervous Debililty

When we think of a kapha person, we usually get a picture of a large, contented individual who oversleeps and does not worry too much. In my practice, however, I have seen people with kapha bodies and aggravated, vata-type minds.

These people are heavy and congested, but may not be able to stop talking. I usually put them on the kapha-pacifying diet to help to break down blockages and *ama* (toxins), but combine this with a vata-pacifying lifestyle for the mind. I recommend more routine and rhythm in their lives, and encourage them to observe more quiet time.

Try the following calming formula for herbal tea:

2 parts skullcap
1 part hops
2 parts passion flower
1 part chamomile
1 part gotu kola
1/2 part rosemary
1/2 part spearmint
1/2 part sage
pinch ginger

Saunas, massage, and exercise may also bring more balance to the kapha person.

Our modern ways are too fast and aggressive. All of us are bombarded with more information than we can possibly assimilate. No matter what our constitutional proclivities may be, everyday life in America is vata-provoking. This must always be taken into consideration.

General Fatigue

Fatigue may be due to many factors and, as with the diagnosis of nervous exhaustion, all lifestyle choices must be reviewed.

Vata Fatigue

Those who display vata imbalances should follow the vata-pacifying diet. The foods must be deeply nourishing and "building." The following herbs, which strengthen the immune system and enhance vitality, may be purchased loose, then cooked into soups, grains, and broths:

Chinese tonic herbs:

1 part astragalus
1 part codonopsis
1 part lychee berries
1 part jujube dates

Put one ounce of this blend into a muslin bag. Place the bag in the pot and cook along with the soup. Remove bag when the food is done. The tasty lychee berries may be added directly to the soup.

Another good formula for the exhausted vata person is the following:

1 part American ginseng
1 part dong quai
1/2 part marshmallow root
1/2 part burdock root
1/4 part licorice root
pinch of ginger

To make tea, simmer one ounce of this blend of herbs 45 minutes in three cups of water. Licorice root has a sweet initial taste and a bitter taste secondarily, so add the licorice root during the last five minutes of cooking. Drink two cups per day, in the morning and afternoon.

Ayurvedic tonic herbs may be blended as follows:

1 tsp. ashwagandha
1 tsp. shatavari
pinch of ginger

Gently simmer these herbs in one cup raw milk or soy milk for 15 minutes. If you are using the powdered herbs, do not strain them. Drink one cup in the morning and another in the afternoon.

Pitta Fatigue

A person with pitta-type fatigue must follow the pitta-pacifying diet and review the lifestyle considerations listed under "Nervous Exhaustion." Due to the burnout they are experiencing, they will also want to add "building" herbs to their foods. For example:

- astragalus
- burdock root
- jujube dates
- lychee berries

Pitta persons may also add to their herbal routine one-half cup aloe vera juice two times per day. Aloe vera juice is a cooling tonic, and is rejuvenative for the liver and spleen. It regulates metabolism of sugar and fat, and tonifies the *agni* (digestive enzymes). It is also excellent for the female reproductive system.

The Ayurvedic herb shatavari may be added to aloe vera juice, or it may be taken in two capsules three times per day. Shatavari is a specific rejuvenative for pitta, for the female reproductive system, and for the blood. It helps to balance women's hormones, and can be used for menopausal women and for those who have had hysterectomies.

A good Western formula for gently rebuilding and detoxifying pitta is:

> Jamaican sarsaparilla
> marshmallow
> burdock root
> nettles
> red clover
> licorice root

Mix together equal parts of the herbs in a jar and add one tablespoon of the combination to a cup of boiling water. Let steep 10 minutes. Drink two or three cups of this tasty tea per day. Or grind the herbs to a powder and put the mixture in "00" capsules; take two capsules three times per day. This formula will remove excess heat from the body, clear the skin of eruptions and nourish the tissues.

Kapha Fatigue

Kapha-type fatigue may be due to excess fat, water, and *ama* (toxins) that block the flow of *prana* (energy). The kapha-pacifying diet must be followed, and an effort must be made not to overeat or sleep after meals. I usually do not give a kapha person or condition strong building herbs such as the ones listed under vata and pitta, because these can increase congestion. Here are some herbal recommendations for the kapha person:

- One-quarter to one-half teaspoon of the trikatu combination (see glossary) may be mixed with honey and taken with meals two or three times per day.

- One-half cup aloe vera juice mixed with a pinch of ginger powder may be taken two times per day.

A combination of the herbs triphala and guggul may be taken in the evening. Put the mixture in "00" capsules and take two at bedtime.

The following Western herbs may be combined and placed in capsules:

2 parts elecampane
1 part kelp
1 part angelica archangelica
1 part dandelion leaf
1/4 part orange peel
1/4 part fennel
1/8 part cayenne

Take two capsules between meals. This formula has many warming and bitter herbs in it, which will help to detoxify accumulated mucus and nourish the tissues. The kelp serves to normalize thyroid function.

Fatigued kaphas should not take strenuous exercise, but ought to make an effort to walk a bit after meals.

Liver Conditions

The liver is considered a "fiery" organ and is the source of most pitta disorders. The word *pitta* means "bile," and excessive bile or a congested bile flow can cause ulcers, heartburn, and other conditions accompanied by burning sensations. There are also many subtle enzymes (called *bhuta agni*) in the liver that help. They digest food particles and help build up tissue for the five sense organs.

The liver is the seat of anger, hate, resentment, jealousy, and ambition, as well as emotions associated with thwarted creativity. When stimulated and unresolved, such emotions can adversely affect the liver. An explosive temper is usually a sign of an overheated liver. The bitter taste promotes the flow of bile, cleanses the blood, detoxifies the liver and thereby relieves an exasperated pitta condition.

Herbs for cleansing and relieving liver heat
- aloe vera juice
- dandelion
- Oregon grape root
- barberry
- goldenseal
- gentian
- yellow dock
- thistle
- bhringaraj
- turmeric
- cyperus

- bupleurum
- gotu kola
- skullcap

Cyperus and bupleurum help to regulate liver energy, aiding digestion and assimilation and regulating mood swings. Gotu kola and skullcap calm the liver and help release us from addictions to substances such as sugar, cigarettes, drugs, and alcohol.

A good combination for relieving the fiery emotions is equal parts:

> skullcap
> passion flower
> gotu kola
> sandalwood

Powder the herbs and take two capsules three times per day, or as needed.

Green leafy vegetables are also good for cleansing the liver. Nettles, beet greens, chickweed, and dandelion leaves contain many vitamins and minerals, and plenty of iron and chlorophyll.

Generally, the person suffering from a liver condition should adhere to the pitta-pacifying diet, avoiding hot spices, acidic foods, fats, oils (except ghee), coffee, black tea, alcohol, and drugs. Many times I recommend that dairy products and meat products be eliminated as well.

Castor oil penetrates deeply into the tissues and gently cleanses the liver. Massage the oil over the whole liver area, just below the rib cage on the right side. If the liver should become "achy," or if you feel that the cleansing is happening too quickly and bringing you discomfort, do not continue using castor oil.

A powerful herb for the liver is seeds of milk thistle, effective against many of the deadly hepatotoxins. Studies have shown that certain milk thistle seed preparations can produce both protective and curative effects when it comes to liver damage resulting from toxic substances. It can be used for various liver diseases, including fatty degeneration of the liver, and can also be supportive treatment for chronic hepatitis and cirrhosis of the liver. I recommend milk thistle seeds in powder or tincture forms, although some herbalists with whom I have spoken sprinkle a tablespoon of the powder on various foods, such as cereals and soups. For liver conditions such as cirrhosis and hepatitis, I do not use alcoholic extracts (tinctures), because the alcohol may exasperate the condition.

Springtime is considered the "liver season," so it is a good idea to pursue a liver-cleansing regime at that time of the year to help detoxify and cleanse out all the winter sludge that may have accumulated. As always, preventative therapy is the best health insurance.

The Gallbladder and Gallstones

The gallbladder is a small gland that presses against the right lobe of the liver and serves as a storage chamber for bile. It releases its contents as needed for the digestion of various substances. When a person has gallstones, they are mainly caused by congestion and obstruction in the flow of bile. Gallstones will often manifest as acute pain in the liver and gallbladder region, and sometimes in the middle-back area. The pain may be accompanied by pronounced inflammation or fever. The herbs for cleansing the liver are appropriate for this condition, with the addition of gravel root, which helps dissolve gallstones.

I have given the following formula to clients with good results:

> 3 parts gravel root
> 1 part dandelion root
> 1 part turmeric root
> 2 parts marshmallow root

> 1/2 part licorice root
> 1/4 part gingerroot

This formula is pain-relieving, detoxifying, and cooling. Take two tablets three times daily; for acute conditions take two tablets every two hours, then decrease the dose as the symptoms subside. Pregnant women should not take this formula.

Gallstones can be quite serious, so make sure that you consult a health practitioner before treating yourself for this condition.

The Woman's "Moon Cycle"

Generally speaking, the way in which a woman's menstrual cycle manifests is a good key into her health situation. In all my sessions with women I ask them about their menstruation—about regularity, discomfort, whether they are or have been on birth control pills, the number of pregnancies, births, or abortions, and so forth. If the menstruation is regular with little pain or tension, and if the emotions do not fluctuate severely each month, these are signs of good health. Most women, however, experience a degree of menstrual discomfort at different times in their lives.

If there has been some imbalance in your cycle, it may take up to four months of regular herbal treatment before you see results. The herbs work slowly to reestablish a new foundation. Be patient and continue on your healing path.

The Vata Woman

The woman with a vata constitution that is out of balance may experience *some* of the following symptoms:
- slow start of menstruation
- brownish blood
- severe cramping and lower-back pain, sometimes lasting for days

- headaches
- chills
- nervousness, anxiety, fear
- difficulty sleeping
- gas and bloating, especially before menstruation
- irregular bowel movements
- short menstruation cycle (two or three days)
- irregular, variable cycle

The patient should follow the vata-pacifying diet, avoiding cold foods and drinks, carbonated drinks, fast foods, and ice cream. The food should be warm and nourishing. Many times excessive exercising, such as aerobics, can deplete the body of needed energy and fluids; it is best for the vata woman to practice yoga or mild exercise instead. An excessively thin person may be deficient in blood as well as energy, which will make for difficult menstruation. Excessive sexual activity can also deplete the vata person of vitality. Just before and during menstruation, observe some quiet time. This will help to calm the mind and nerves.

During menstruation, most women become introspective. Introspection helps us to be more in tune with our inner voice and vision. Do not be afraid of this inner journey. Instead, learn to see it as a companion to self-realization.

Nourishing tonic herbs for the vata woman
- dong quai
- vitex
- rehmannia
- licorice root
- shatavari
- ashwagandha
- comfrey root
- wild yam root

- marshmallow root
- saw palmetto

Shatavari (*asparagus racemosus*) is one of the best-known Ayurvedic herbs for the female reproductive system, nourishing, calming the heart, and demulcent for dry and inflamed membranes of the lungs, stomach, kidneys, and sexual organs. Shatavari nourishes and cleanses the blood and the reproductive organs. It can be used for menopause and for those who have had hysterectomies. It is sattvic in quality, promoting love and devotion.

Although some Ayurvedic practitioners believe that ashwagandha (*withania somnifera*) is an herb for the male system, I have used it many times, in combination with other tonic herbs, for the female system. Ashwagandha is a rejuvenative herb for the vata constitution, working in particular on the muscles, marrow, and reproductive system. It is good for all conditions of weakness and deficiency. I have had excellent results using it with pregnant women, and also with children who are weak. Try the following formula:

2 parts shatavari
2 parts ashwagandha
1 part vitex
1 part licorice root
1/4 part ginger
Take two "00" capsules three times per day with meals.

Dong quai (*angelica sinensis*) is used in the treatment of many female gynecological ailments. It regulates menstruation, tonifies the blood, promotes blood circulation, and counteracts dryness of the bowels that causes constipation. It should not be used by pregnant women or those suffering from wasting diseases, or when there is bloating, abdominal congestion, or uterine fibroids. Dong quai's phyto-estrogenic qualities make it helpful for the menopausal woman as well.

Here is another simple formula:
2 parts dong quai
1 part vitex
1 part wild yam
2 parts licorice root
1/8 part ginger
Take two "00" capsules three times per day with meals.

For cramps

1 part cramp bark
1 part pennyroyal
1 part valerian
1 part blue cohosh
1/2 part ginger

Put about one tablespoon each of cramp bark and blue cohosh, in a quart of boiling water. Let simmer for 20 minutes. Turn the heat off and add one tablespoon each of valerian, pennyroyal, and 1/2 teaspoon ginger. You do not want to boil these last three herbs, as the essential oils and active ingredients will dissipate. Let them steep for an additional 20 minutes. Drink 1/4 to 1/2 cup every 15–30 minutes until you experience some relief.

A ginger foot bath may be helpful as well, stimulating the flow of blood and warming up the system. Put one tablespoon of powdered ginger in a small tub and add warm water. Let your feet soak for 15 or more minutes, adding hot water as needed. A hot compress of ginger tea may be placed against the uterus as well.

The Pitta Woman

If the pitta woman is out of balance, then *some* of the following symptoms may occur:

- loose stool before menstruation
- feelings of irritation and anger

- heavy bleeding with some clotting
- achy breasts (due to liver congestion)
- painful cramping
- rashes, acne, or herpes outbreaks
- excess heat, night sweats, or hot flashes
- headaches
- redness of the eyes

The pitta-pacifying diet should be followed, with strict avoidance of acidic foods such as oranges and tomatoes. Hot spices, alcohol, coffee, and excess meats should be excluded from the diet. Sunbathing and saunas also may overheat the pitta woman.

Tonic herbs for the pitta woman
- aloe vera juice
- shatavari
- vitex
- sarsaparilla
- wild yam
- dong quai (high doses may aggravate pitta)
- black cohosh
- licorice root
- peony root

Cooling astringent herbs for toning the uterus
- nettles
- raspberry leaves
- motherwort
- strawberry leaves
- squaw vine

The liver herbs are important for the pitta person as well. They will keep the energy flowing and help to alleviate some of the anger, heat, and frustration that may manifest. The liver also helps to process many of the hormones in the body, thus easing menstruation.

Here's a good tonic formula for the pitta woman:

2 parts wild yam
2 parts licorice
1 part burdock root
2 parts dandelion root
1 part comfrey root
2 parts sarsaparilla
1 part vitex
1/2 part dong quai
1/4 part ginger

Powder the herbs and take two "00" capsules three times per day.

Try out this tasty tea:

2 parts raspberry leaf
2 parts nettles
1 part spearmint
1 part lemongrass

Put one tablespoon of the combination in a cup of boiling water and let it steep for 10 minutes. Strain and drink two or three cups per day.

The herb motherwort may be used for night sweats and hot flashes. It is also good for heart palpitations. This herb is quite bitter, so I usually use it in tincture form.

For Cramping

2 parts chamomile (Note: people who are allergic to ragweed may be allergic to chamomile)
1 part yarrow
1 part cramp bark
1 part skullcap
1 part peppermint
1 part squaw vine

Gently simmer the cramp bark for 10 minutes, then add the other herbs and steep together for an additional 10 minutes. Strain and drink 1/4 cup every 15 minutes until some relief is felt. A hot ginger compress placed against the uterus may also be helpful.

The Kapha Woman

The kapha woman who is out of balance may have *some* of the following symptoms:

- water retention
- mucus in the blood
- mucus in the stool or urine
- feelings of heaviness and tiredness
- excess saliva and phlegm
- breasts swollen due to water retention
- teary sentimental feelings
- food feels heavy in the stomach
- nausea
- excess or emotional eating
- mild cramping with a "heavy" feeling

Follow the kapha-pacifying diet, strictly avoiding dairy, ice cream, sweets, fatty fried foods, oils, nuts, and salt. Make sure that each meal is fully digested before consuming more food. Do not drink too many liquids.

Spices such as cayenne and trikatu (see glossary) will help to stimulate the metabolism, thus relieving congestion and water retention. Another formula that works with the kidney to eliminate excess water is:

2 parts dandelion leaves
2 parts cleavers
1 part chickweed
1 part uva ursi

Take three "00" capsules three times per day, or drink

three cups of tea per day. To make a tea, take one tablespoon of the herb blend and let it steep in a cup of boiling water until it cools to room temperature.

The herbs for the liver are appropriate for the kapha woman, and should be taken 15 minutes before meals.

Tonic Herbs for the Kapha Woman
- dong quai (*angelica sinensis*)
- angelica archangelica
- black cohosh
- blue cohosh
- aloe vera juice
- false unicorn
- ashwagandha
- wild yam
- damiana

For Cramping
- blue cohosh
- black cohosh
- ginger
- "cramp bark"
- chamomile

Astringent herbs for toning the uterus
- motherwort
- raspberry leaves
- nettles
- strawberry leaves

Spices should be added to the diet, and as well as to the formulas for the kapha person. One of the actions of the spicy or pungent taste is to counteract stagnation and increase blood circulation. Many of the common spices, such as turmeric, cinnamon, ginger, cayenne, basil, cardamom, asafoetida, garlic, fennel, and dill, can be used for delayed or slowed menstruation, and also to alleviate cramping.

Here is a simple but effective formula for nourishing the reproductive organs in the kapha individual:

2 parts dong quai
2 parts wild yam
1 part burdock root
2 parts dandelion root
1 part vitex
1/2 part ginger

Take two "00" capsules or one dropperful of the tincture three times per day.

Elimination, Tonification, and Rejuvenation

When we consider implementing an herbal program, we must decide whether the case calls for *eliminating* toxins or for *building* tissues, blood, or energy.

Elimination therapies focus on decreasing weight, accumulated ama (toxins), and excess humors. In Ayurveda, this type of therapy is called *langhana*, which literally means "to lighten."

When a person has an acute condition such as a cold, flu, or cough, eliminating therapies are employed. Elimination methods include:

- sweating techniques using saunas and diaphoretic herbs
- clearing the bowels with herbs that have a laxative action (purgatives)
- elimination through the urine (diuretic herbs)
- elimination through vomiting (emetic herbs)
- eliminating phlegm from the lungs (expectorants)
- discharging of gas (carminative herbs)
- destroying pathogens with blood-, lymph- and bile-cleansing herbs (alterative herbs)

These techniques can also be used as part of a disease-prevention and internal-cleansing program to eliminate deep-seated toxins. Especially during the transitional seasons of spring and fall, it is good to undergo a light fast and cleansing program to help eliminate toxins and accumulated humors which may otherwise cause difficulties.

Tonification or supplementation therapy uses herbs and foods that build, nourish, and strengthen tissues. In Ayurveda this is call *brimhana*, meaning "to make heavy." Tonification is indicated for individuals who are elderly, malnourished, chronically ill, pregnant, emaciated, convalescent, anemic, infertile, impotent, or suffering from nervous exhaustion and emotional collapse. It is also helpful in cases of chronic insomnia.

Some tonic herbs increase the energy and vitality of the organ systems by providing deeply nourishing vitamins, minerals, and sugars. Others act to balance the energy of the organs, improving their ability to assimilate nutrients. The rule of thumb is to first eliminate toxins, then tonify. If we try to tonify while there is still accumulated ama in the system, the tonic herbs may actually exacerbate the condition. A short fast, a series of saunas, and consumption of blood-cleansing herbs can help reduce toxins and make the tonifying therapy more effective.

A tonic is most effective taken with food. Herbs such as ginseng, astragalus, dong quai, codonopsis, and shatavari may be simmered in soups. The famous Ayurvedic formula chyavanprash combines more than 25 finely powdered herbs in a base of honey and ghee to make a delicious paste.

Other tonic herbs include:

Chinese herbs:

- panax ginseng
- Siberian ginseng
- codonopsis
- astragalus
- atractylodes
- rehmannia
- peony root
- ho shou wu

Ayurvedic herbs:

- shatavari
- triphala

- ashwagandha
- kapikacchu
- amalaki

Others:
- licorice root
- American ginseng
- marshmallow root
- comfrey root
- elecampane
- false unicorn
- damiana
- saw palmetto
- aloe vera
- suma
- garlic
- solomon's seal
- slippery elm
- ophiopogon

Vata Tonification Therapy

Vata requires the strongest tonifying therapies, all in the context of plenty of rest, oil massage, and warm baths with mineral salts. Heavy exercising, excess sexual activity, too much talking, and the stress of travel all disperse energy and therefore should be avoided. Instead, provide a quiet environment and nourishing foods.

Tonic herbs specific for vata include:
- shatavari
- marshmallow
- comfrey root
- saw palmetto
- kapikacchu
- triphala

- astragalus
- dong quai
- Siberian ginseng
- American ginseng
- ashwagandha
- ophiopogon
- guggul (Note: guggul is not a nutritive tonic in it-self, but helps to catalyze tissue regeneration, particularly of the nerve tissue, reducing toxins, increasing white-blood cell count, and helping with conditions of arthritis, gout, nervous disorders, diabetes, obesity, and skin disease. It is particularly good for vata and kapha, but will aggravate pitta if taken in large doses over a long period of time. Taken alone it may be too harsh in its action, so it is usually mixed with other herbs.)

Mild spices may be used with the formulas and in the food. These include:
- ginger
- cinnamon
- cloves
- asafoetida
- fennel
- dill
- rosemary

Pitta Tonification Therapy

The tonification therapy for pitta is moderate compared to that of vata. Mild massage is fine, but without the use of too much oil. Saunas, hot tubs, and sweat lodges should be avoided. Warm baths and showers are fine. Jogging in the middle of the day, strenuous aerobics, and heavy weight-lifting should be replaced with mild exercises and yoga. The pitta-pacifying diet should be adhered to, but with more of the building foods and herbs. Raw foods and juices should be kept to a minimum.

Tonic herbs for pitta include:
- amalaki
- shatavari
- marshmallow root
- gotu kola
- rehmannia
- licorice
- aloe vera
- peony root
- ho shou wu
- Siberian ginseng

Pitta should avoid hot spices, alcohol, coffee, and other stimulants. The lifestyle should be free from competition and aggression, which will reduce vitality.

Kapha Tonification Therapy

The tonification therapy for kapha is more stimulating than building. Moderate-strength massage and mild sweating therapy are fine. Adequate rest should be taken, but do not sleep after meals or during the day. Exercise should be mild, such as walking or gently jumping on an exercise trampoline.

The kapha-pacifying diet should be followed, but with an emphasis on the more building foods. Raw foods, cold foods, dairy products, and excess oils should be avoided.

Good tonic herbs for kapha include:
- elecampane
- guggul
- aloe vera with spices
- garlic
- saffron
- angelica archangelica

- dong quai
- gotu kola
- triphala

Spices may be used in the formulas and foods to help counteract stagnation, but not in excess.

Pancha Karma and Rejuvenation

Pancha karma consists of five very intensive and radical cleansing techniques employed in Ayurveda—not just the application of the elimination methods discussed earlier, but an intensive system for guiding the toxins to specific sites for elimination. The five techniques are:

1. therapeutic vomiting
2. purgation
3. enemas
4. nasal application of herbs
5. therapeutic release of toxic blood

Prior to pancha karma, preliminary techniques called *purva karma* are employed. These consist of application of oil, followed by steam or therapeutic sweating therapy. The oils help to loosen and liquify the ama and humors in the skin and blood. They eventually drain into the gastrointestinal tract, where they are eliminated by the pancha karma techniques listed above.

Rejuvenation therapy, or *rasayana*, is a special type of tonification that follows pancha karma. The herbs and application are the same as for tonification therapy, but are applied in a manner calculated to bring about an energized and revitalized new person. It is beyond the capacity of this small booklet to explain these techniques in any detail. For further information, please consult one or more of the resources listed at the end of this book.

Case Studies—Ayurveda in Action

Case #1: Ken

Ken came to see me with a severe condition of ulcerated colitis, from which he had been suffering for fifteen years. He was forty-five years old, tall, medium build, dark hair, with pock-marked skin from acne, intense dark eyes, and a gentle manner. He liked to talk and was very free in describing to me his history and situation.

While a soldier in Vietnam, he had been introduced to marijuana and heroin. For five years he was a heroin addict. He had also been a heavy drinker. At one point he had kidney failure due to an overdose of heroin, and currently had a cyst on one kidney. At 28 years of age he went into a recovery house and began to eliminate drugs and alcohol from his life. He was drug- and alcohol-free when he came to see me.

His symptoms were classically those of provoked pitta (fire element). He ached in the liver and gallbladder area, while experiencing burning sensations in the digestive tract. His stools were loose and hot. He did not sleep well and felt agitated. From time to time, he had blood in the stool and suffered from hemorrhoids. He also had chronic hepatitis with a high liver-enzyme count. He was currently on disability, and was not employed or in retraining. He never came down with acute ailments such as colds or flus.

Ken's diet was quite poor. He started the day off with two cups of coffee with Sweet and Low. During the day he ate just a little fruit, mostly apples and bananas, and in the evening he would eat some rice or a very light meal. I was astonished that he still had the energy to bike for 10 miles each day and still do some work around the house.

His pulse on the right wrist was strong, more a "jumping" pitta pulse. The pulse on the left hand was indiscernible due to the collapse of blood vessels that occurred during drug use.

When viewing his tongue I saw many red lines in the very back section, which indicates a heated condition of the intestines and colon. The sides of the tongue, which show the liver and gallbladder, were red, and the tongue was swollen as well.

Ken, I could see, was suffering from a condition of overall inflammation, which is pitta in nature. The stool was loose, excessively flowing, sharp (burning sensation), excessively liquid, and there was an aggressive and penetrating character to the condition.

The first obvious thing about this case was that Ken needed to stop drinking coffee, which tends to disperse energy and stimulate the nervous system, including the peristaltic action of the bowels. The seventeen alkaloids in coffee, which must be processed by the liver, strain that organ's functions. Coffee is also quite acidic, and will eat away at the mucous lining of the digestive tract.

I had Ken take amalaki, two capsules with water, each night before bed. (Amalaki is a bowel regulator for pittas and colitis. It gently cleanses the liver and kidneys, and helps regulate metabolism.) Three nights a week I had Ken rub the liver and colon area with castor oil, which penetrates deeply into the tissues, and helps cleanse the liver and heal tissue.

I also gave him a bitter formula with milk thistle seeds (two capsules 15 minutes before meals) to help detoxify the liver and protect it as well. The main formula for the ulcerated colitis was:

3 parts agrimony
2 parts wild yam

2 parts goldenseal
1 part marshmallow
1 part bayberry

Three capsules were to be taken three times per day before meals. This formula is specific for healing ulcerations of the digestive tract, calming spasms, staunching bleeding and reinstating healthy mucus in the tract lining.

Ken was already taking flaxseed oil, vitamin C, acidophilus and psyllium. I told him to continue with these supplements.

When Ken called me a couple of weeks later, he told me that he had not stopped drinking coffee and that the colitis situation had worsened. He asked what other herbs he should take, but I insisted that the herbs would work as soon as he stopped the coffee intake. He called me again about six weeks later and thanked me for the advice. The diarrhea and bleeding had ceased about 10 days after he stopped drinking coffee. So had the symptoms of colitis. He was eating a much healthier, pitta-pacifying diet and had gained weight. He said that he felt so good that he was on a retraining program with a local college and had acquired a new girlfriend.

This example shows how important it is to address the dietary choices that the person is making. Herbs have a hard time working if the diet is counter to the treatment.

Case #2: Cheryl

Cheryl is one of my regular clients and has come to see me many times over the past six years. She is forty-eight years old, slender, small build, and has a tendency to feel cold in winter and comfortable in the summer. She has been very conscious of her food and lifestyle choices, and eats quite healthily. She has a long-term, stable relationship with her spouse and enjoys her employment as a social worker.

Her constitution is vata-pitta, with vata slightly higher than pitta. During the winter through early spring she follows the vata-pacifying diet with mostly cooked foods, extra spices and tonifying, building herbs. In the summer she has a tendency to overheat, so she follows the pitta-pacifying diet during the very hot months.

Cheryl is in excellent health generally, but came to me complaining of headaches that occurred in the morning when she woke up, and also in the afternoon. She said she was sleeping well, with no insomnia or restlessness. We went over her diet and the herbs she was taking on a regular basis, and could not find anything that stood out as a possible cause of the headaches.

I had Cheryl describe to me the room she slept in and learned that the window was open all night and always let in a cool breeze, right at her head. At work she had a similar situation: the air vent was right over her and would cool her head all day. I told Cheryl to close the bedroom window at night and open another window that did not blow directly onto her.

The situation at work was trickier. She first tried to tilt the air vent so that it did not blow directly onto her. This proved difficult to accomplish, so I suggested she wear a hat or scarf, and that she wrap a small blanket around the kidney area and use a heating pad if her feet grew cold. I told her to report back to me after a couple of weeks.

The headaches stopped immediately upon changing the environments. She called again a few months later and said that she was still headache-free. The air vent and open window tended to create a cold, dry, mobile, agitating, and dispersing atmosphere, provoking a vata-type headache.

Looking at this example, we see that it is important to not only look at the diet and foods, but also the patient's environment.

Case #3: Susan

The next case was quite complicated. Susan, 42, had many chronic conditions that had begun to culminate in a general loss of vitality. She felt it had started three years earlier, when she had a knee operation following an injury. She had been given dozens of different anesthetics, gone into shock, and almost died. She had lost 20 pounds and felt that she had never got over that trauma.

Upon questioning her further, I found out that Susan had once suffered from colitis, which had stopped five years ago after she cut coffee out of her diet. In recent months the colitis had flared up again, but seemed to be under control now—although her stool continued to be runny.

Susan also had manifested some unusual conditions from birth. Her mother had taken different drug therapies to help with the pregnancy. The drugs created in Susan a double uterus, an appendix on the wrong side of the body, and one weak kidney. Susan also suffered from stomach bloating, arthritis of the left hand, anxiety attacks, shortness of breath, heart palpitations, allergies, eczema, and vaginal yeast. She was currently on birth control pills, Motrin for arthritis pain, and antihistamines. She had recently started on wheat grass juice and antioxidant vitamins.

Susan is medium build with light hair, skin, and eyes, a very driven person with great ambition and willpower. Her pulse was quite weak, but had a slight "jumping" quality to it. Her tongue was very red on the sides, indicating heat in the liver and gallbladder. The back of the tongue had a yellow coating, indicating heat in the lower part of her body, probably the intestines and colon.

I felt that Susan's prakruti (basic constitution) was predominantly pitta, with secondary vata and kapha (i.e., V2-P3-K1) Her vikruti (current condition) was V3-P4-K1. Vata and pitta were both elevated. Among the conditions that definitely pointed to vata were the anxiety, the palpitations, arthritis, and the shortness of breath. The pitta-provoked conditions were the colitis, the vaginal infection and the allergies.

I put Susan on the pitta-pacifying diet, but with an emphasis on the vata-pacifying lifestyle. Her meals were to be taken at regular hours and never skipped. She was to go to bed no later than 10 p.m. and was to use sesame oil on her feet, mixed with lavender essential oil for calming. She was not to watch the news or read anything that aroused turbulent emotions. I even had her make an herbal pillow stuffed with herbs for calming, such as chamomile, lemon balm, hops, lavender, and rose petals.

I had Susan cut out all alcohol from her diet, along with white sugar, all dairy, and any yeasted breads. (These foods would increase her yeast condition.) She was to take an acidophilus supplement three times per day to reinstate the good flora which had been destroyed by the drugs, antibiotics, and birth control pills.

If Susan experienced a vaginal infection, she was to do the following:

- Make a strong tea with 1/2 teaspoon goldenseal to one cup boiling water. Steep for 30 minutes and strain. Douche with this tea once per day for up to three days.
- Follow each douche with a second douche containing one teaspoon acidophilus powder to reinstate the good flora in the vaginal region.

The doctor had told her to ice her arthritic hand each day, but this was just stopping the flow of healing blood to the area. I instructed her in using what Chinese medicine calls "moxibustion," a method of burning herbs, such as mugwort, above the skin to warm the area and thus break down blockages. It is wonderful for sprains, injuries, and arthritis. Many times pain is due to blockage, and in Susan's case the arthritis was a definite area of congestion. I also instructed her to put some warming liniment on the area following the moxibustion.

For Susan's liver, I put together a bitter formula to help in detoxification. I did not give her any alcoholic extract, however, because I felt that the alcohol would exacerbate the situation. All the formulas were taken in capsules or teas.

In the evening before bed, Susan was to take two capsules of amalaki, and one of the herbs in the triphala compound, which is excellent for bleeding disorders, colitis, palpitations, and general debility, and is rejuvenative for pitta as well. She also was to take one-half cup of aloe vera juice two times per day.

I also gave her an arthritis formula containing:

yucca
black cohosh
white willow bark
marshmallow root
guggul (a special Ayurvedic resin for scraping toxins from the tissues)
angelica archangelica
licorice root
ginger

She took two capsules three times per day.

For a relaxing beverage tea, I mixed together the following nervines:

passion flower
lemon balm
skullcap
hops
rose petals
spearmint
lavender
chamomile

She was to drink one cup 30 minutes before bedtime.

Susan called me about a month after the session and reported that her arthritic hand was much better. She was able to work at the computer without much discomfort and was down to only one Motrin per week. She no longer suffered from anxiety attacks and was able to sleep quite well most nights. Her stools were solid and regular now, and the vaginal infection had not recurred.

She returned to work full-time, which has been a strain on her, but today she rests during her times off and believes she knows how to conduct her life in such a way that the healing process will continue.

Case #4: Bill

Bill, 48, had been suffering from a mucousy, irritating cough for about six months. It had started off as a severe cold during the winter, for which he had been prescribed antibiotics. His symptoms were worse at night and in the morning. His doctor wanted to prescribe a daily dose of antibiotics for an indefinite period of time. His digestion was poor, with a heavy feeling after meals, along with more mucus in the throat area.

After talking to Bill, I determined that his prakruti was V1-P3-K2. However, kapha was provoked at this time and stood at 3. Because he reported seeing mucus in the stool, as well as in the nasal area, I believed that the mucus had settled not only in the lungs, but throughout his system.

Some of the qualities of kapha are:
- cold
- damp
- heavy
- liquid
- thick
- slow

Bill was chilly most of the time, and his lungs and sinuses felt cool and damp. The mucus was thick and white, and tended to be heavy in texture. Bill felt heavy after eating and needed to rest more often than usual. All these symptoms pointed to a kapha condition. (Bill did not have any heat or burning symptoms, nor did he have any dryness or vata conditions, so I did not feel that the vata or pitta part of his constitution was provoked at this time.)

I put Bill on the kapha-pacifying diet with an emphasis on spices and warm foods. I told him to stop taking ice water and other cold drinks, which create mucus. He also was to eliminate all dairy, fatty foods, nuts, and oils. This was his program:

1. Bill was to start the day off with a dry body brushing with a loofa sponge or vegetable fiber brush. This would stimulate the lymphatic system and help to release congestion and toxins.

2. In the morning and evening, he was to do a nasal wash with one teaspoon of sea salt per cup of warm water.

3. He was to take a milk-free acidophilus supplement, two capsules three times per day, to reinstate the good flora that had been killed off by the antibiotic therapy.

4. He was to take bitters 15 minutes before meals; after meals, he was to take one-half teaspoon of trikatu paste (see glossary).

5. He was to take two capsules of triphala each night before bed to help regulate the bowels and cleanse the colon, liver, and kidneys.

6. The main formula for the lungs was:

> 2 parts elecampane
> 1 part grindelia
> 1 part marshmallow root
> 1 part horehound
> 1/2 part wild cherry bark
> 1/4 part lobelia
> 1/4 part ginger
> 1/4 part goldenseal

7. He was to drink ginger tea and other spicy beverages throughout the day, and avoid cold drinks.

Because Bill worked long hours each day, we decided that capsules would be most convenient. He took two "00" capsules three times per day on an empty stomach. I told him to take a cup of tea with the herbs listed in number 6 at least once per day, preferably in the morning. He let one tablespoon of the herbs steep in hot water overnight so that all he had to do in the morning was strain and reheat it.

Within three weeks the coughing bouts had stopped; there was just a little residual mucus in the nasal area upon waking. We changed the formula a bit, eliminating the lobelia, goldenseal, and wild cherry bark, and added some bayberry and a little cayenne. He was soon symptom-free.

In this example we see how an illness may reflect a condition different from your basic constitution. Bill was predominantly a pitta person, but his pitta was not aggravated; it was kapha that had been provoked. In Ayurveda it is said that it is easier to cure a condition that is different than your basic constitution, because the basic constitution is not reinforcing the illness.

Appendix 1: Aromatherapy for the Three Doshas

Essential oils, used most often as perfumes or as fragrances for massage oils, may help to open the heart center and to allay negative emotions such as fear, irritation, and apathy.

For a massage oil, mix together 15 to 20 drops of essential oil (your choice) in four ounces of almond oil and shake well. For an atomizer or other spray bottle, add 15 to 20 drops of essential oil to four ounces of distilled water, and shake well.

"Candle burners," available at health food stores, are very popular as well. Place 10 drops of essential oil into the bowl of water and light the candle below it. A light fragrance will pervade into the air, creating the desired effect.

Caution: applying essential oils directly to the skin may cause severe skin damage. Taking them internally can be extremely dangerous, and may cause death. (One ounce of essential oil is equivalent in potency to thirty two bathtubs of strong herb tea.) Unless you have studied with an aromatherapist, use the essential oils only as suggested above. And make sure that you purchase essential oils, not "fragrances," which are made from synthetic ingredients and do not carry the same health benefits.

Essential Oils for Vata
- jasmine
- sandalwood
- lavender
- rose geranium

- fennel
- pine
- camphor
- frankincense
- basil
- cinnamon
- cardamom
- orange
- angelica

These aromas are calming, warming, and grounding.

Essential Oils for Pitta
- sandalwood
- lavender
- rose geranium
- orange
- lemongrass
- fennel
- peppermint
- jasmine
- gardenia
- mints
- vetiver

These aromas are cooling, calming, and peace-inducing.

Essential Oils for Kapha
- camphor
- cedar
- cinnamon
- frankincense
- cloves
- myrrh
- musk
- pennyroyal

- thyme
- mugwort
- lemongrass
- basil
- lavender
- juniper
- rosemary
- sage

These aromas are stimulating and energizing.

Appendix 2: Color Therapy for Vata, Pitta, Kapha

Vata Colors

Warm, soft shades of:
- red
- gold
- orange
- yellow

Combining these colors with moist and calm colors, such as white or light shades of green or blue, can be very good for vata. Too-bright colors, such as flashy reds or purples, will aggravate the nervous sensitivity of vata types or vata conditions.

Under certain conditions, dark colors may be grounding for vata.

Pitta Colors
- white
- blue
- green
- pastels

Colors that are hot, sharp, or stimulating, like red, orange, and yellow, will aggravate pitta and pitta conditions. Very bright or iridescent colors will provoke pitta. Pastels of various shades are fine.

Kapha Colors

Bright shades of:
- yellow
- gold
- red
- orange

Kaphas can wear bright shades with lots of color contrasts. White, pink, or light shades of "cool" colors such as blue and green are not good for kaphas, although very bright or brilliant shades of blue and green are recommended.

Glossary

agni: "digestive fires," i.e., secretions of the digestive system that help break down undigested food (*ama*) and release energy.

ama: undigested food material that becomes lodged in the body's weakest organs and may precipitate disease conditions.

Ayurveda: the science and wisdom of life. *Ayur* means "life" or "longevity"; *veda* means "knowledge" or "wisdom."

brimhana: a tonifying therapy that uses herbs and foods to build, nourish, and strengthen tissues.

dosha: the Sanskrit word for "humor," or one of the three biological forces that bind the five elements into living flesh. They are known as vata, pitta, and kapha. Literally translated, dosha means "that which darkens, spoils, or causes things to decay." When out of balance, the doshas (humors) are the causative forces in the disease process. In balance, they create a healthy and harmonious body.

ghee: clarified butter. Excellent for digestion. To prepare ghee, use a medium to heavy saucepan. Melt at a very low temperature one pound of unsalted butter. (Organic and/or raw is best, if available.) The butter will make bubbling sounds as foam forms on the top. Stir in the foam and continue to cook the ghee. If you look at the bottom of the pan, you will notice milk solids forming. You will notice also that the butter no longer bubbles. (The process takes about 30 minutes or so, depending on your stove.) Take the ghee off the burner as soon as it has stopped bubbling and is clear-looking. Let it cool a bit, then pour it through a metal strainer into a glass jar. Discard the milk solids that are stuck on the bottom of the pan. Ghee will store at room temperature.

gunas: the three attributes (*sattva*, *rajas* and *tamas*) that are the foundation of all existence.

kapha: one of the three *doshas* (humors) of the body; it has the qualities of water and earth.

langhana: a "lightening" therapy that focuses on effecting a decrease in weight, accumulated toxins, and excess humors.

lassi: A nourishing drink made from fresh plain yogurt, water, and spices, often served at the end of a meal as a digestive aid.

Mildly Spicy Lassi Drink

1/2 cup plain yogurt
2 cups pure water
1/4 tsp. powdered ginger
1/4 tsp. cumin powder
1/8 tsp. salt

Blend all ingredients for a few minutes. Drink at room temperature, 1/4 to 1/2 cup after meals. May be garnished with cilantro leaves.

Sweet Lassi

1/2 cup plain fresh yogurt
2 cups pure water
2 tbsp. natural sugar (Sucanat®, barley malt, etc.; add less
sweetener for kaphas)
1/4 tsp. dry ginger
1/2 tsp. ground cardamom
1/4 tsp. cinnamon
Blend together for a few minutes. Drink at room
temperature, 1/4 to 1/2 cup after meals.

ojas: the subtle essence of all the kapha, or water, in the body.
Ojas is the prime energy reserve in the body, and the vitality of
the immune system.

pancha karma: the five radical cleansing techniques employed
in Ayurveda.

pitta: one of the three *doshas* (humors) of the body; it has the
qualities of fire and water.

prana: the life force, called *chi* in Oriental medicine.

prakruti: fixed proportions of vata, pitta, kapha established at
conception; inherited nature; also, the principle of creativity
or primal nature.

purva karma: various milder treatments used as a preliminary
to *pancha karma*.

purusha: the absolute, unmanifested state of consciousness.

rajas: the cosmic force of action and activity; in the mind, rajas creates aggression and overactivity.

rasayana: Ayurvedic rejuvenation therapy, a special type of tonification.

sattva: the cosmic force of balance and equilibrium; helps to maintain clarity of mind.

Sucanat®: a natural sugar made from organic sugar-cane juice, containing all its inherent minerals and vitamins.

tamas: the cosmic force of inactivity and inertia; in the mind, tamas creates dullness and resistance to change and growth.

tri-dosha: the three bodily humors or constitutions: vata, pitta, kapha.

trikatu: a combination of powdered ginger, black pepper, and pippali pepper. Equal amounts of these herbs are mixed together, with raw honey added to create a paste. One-quarter to one-half teaspoon may be taken with meals or after meals to facilitate digestion. The pippali pepper may be hard to find, so powdered anise seeds may be substituted. This formula is also very good for breaking up mucus.

vata: one of the three *doshas* (humors) of the body; vata has the qualities of air and space.

vikruti: the current state of your health and well-being, as opposed to the fixed state, or *prakruti*.

Recommended Reading and Resources

Books

The following books are particularly useful to beginning students of the Ayurvedic path:

Ayurvedic Healing by Dr. David Frawley; Passage Press, Salt Lake City, Utah 1989.

The Yoga of Herbs by Dr. David Frawley and Dr. Vasant Lad; Lotus Press, Twin Lakes, Wisconsin, 1986.

Ayurvedic Cookbook for Self-Healing by Dr. Vasant Lad; Ayurvedic Press, Albuquerque, New Mexico 1994.

Ayurveda: The Science of Self-Healing by Dr. Vasant Lad; Lotus Press, Twin Lakes, Wisconsin 1985.

The Ayurvedic Cookbook by Amadea Morningstar; Lotus Press, Twin Lakes, Wisconsin 1990.

Ayurveda Beauty Care by Melanie Sachs; Lotus Press, Twin Lakes, Wisconsin, 1992.

Ayurveda: Life, Health and Longevity by Rob Svoboda; Arkana, Toronto, Canada 1992.

Prakruti: Your Ayurvedic Constitution by Rob Svoboda; Geocom, New Mexico 1988.

Planetary Herbology by Dr. Michael Tierra; Lotus Press, Twin Lakes, Wisconsin 1988.

The Way of Herbs by Dr. Michael Tierra; Simon and Schuster, New York, New York 1980.

Ayurveda: A Life of Balance by Maya Tiwari; Healing Arts Press, Rochester, Vermont 1995.

Ayurvedic Studies

EverGreen Herb Garden
(intensive study programs, incorporating herbology and Ayurveda)
Candis Cantin Packard
P.O. Box 1445
Placerville, CA 95667
(916) 626-9288
Call or write for information.

American Institute of Vedic Studies
Dr. David Frawley
Ayurvedic Correspondence Course
P.O. Box 8357
Santa Fe, NM 87504

The Ayurvedic Institute
(nine-month study program)
Dr. Vasant Lad
P.O. Box 23445
Albuquerque, NM 87192-1445

Aromatherapy Oils

Leydet Oils
P.O. Box 2354
Fair Oaks, CA 95628
Write for brochure.

Ayurvedic Herbs

Bazaar of India
(wholesale and retail)
1810 University Ave.
Berkeley, CA 94703
Write for brochure.
(800) 261-SOMA

Lotus Light
(wholesale)
P.O. Box 1008, Dept. ABC
Silver Lake, WI 53170
(414) 889-8501

Chinese Herbs

May Way Trading Co.
622 Broadway
San Francisco, CA 94133
(415) 788-3646

Western Herbs and Products

Mountain Rose Herbs
P.O. Box 2000
Redway, CA 95560
(800) 879-3337

Trinity Herb Company
P.O. Box 199
Bodega, CA 94922
(707) 874-3418

Index

(For definition of italicized items, see Glossary)

The Crossing Press publishes a full
selection of titles on alternative
health and healing. To receive our
current catalog, please call toll-free,
1-800-777-1048